Visual Impairment:
A Global View

Introducing Health Sciences: A Case Study Approach

Series editor: Basiro Davey

Seven case studies on major topics in global public health are the subject of this multidisciplinary series of books, each with its own animations, videos and learning activities on DVD. They focus on: access to clean water in an overcrowded and polluted world; the integration of psychological and biological approaches to pain; alcohol consumption and its effects on the body; the science, risks and benefits of mammography screening for early breast cancer; chronic lung disease due to smoke pollution – a forgotten cause of millions of deaths worldwide; traffic-related injuries, tissue repair and recovery; and the causes and consequences of visual impairment in developed and developing countries. Each topic integrates biology, chemistry, physics and psychology with health statistics and social studies to illuminate the causes of disease and disability, their impacts on individuals and societies and the science underlying common treatments. These case studies will be of value to anyone who is, or wants to be, working in a health-related occupation where scientific knowledge could enhance your prospects. If you have a wide-ranging interest in human sciences and want to learn more about global health issues and statistics, how the body works and the scientific rationale for screening procedures and treatments, this series is for you.

Titles in this series

Water and Health in an Overcrowded World, edited by Tim Halliday and Basiro Davey

Pain, edited by Frederick Toates

Alcohol and Human Health, edited by Lesley Smart

Screening for Breast Cancer, edited by Elizabeth Parvin

Chronic Obstructive Pulmonary Disease: A Forgotten Killer, edited by Carol Midgley

Trauma, Repair and Recovery, edited by James Phillips

Visual Impairment: A Global View, edited by Heather McLannahan

Visual Impairment:
A Global View

Edited by Heather McLannahan

 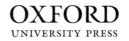

Published by Oxford University Press, Great Clarendon Street, Oxford OX2 6DP
in association with The Open University, Walton Hall, Milton Keynes MK7 6AA.

OXFORD
UNIVERSITY PRESS

Oxford University Press is a department of the University of Oxford. It furthers the University's
objective of excellence in research, scholarship, and education by publishing worldwide in

Oxford New York

Auckland Cape Town Dar es Salaam Hong Kong Karachi Kuala Lumpur Madrid Melbourne
Mexico City Nairobi New Delhi Shanghai Taipei Toronto

with offices in

Argentina Austria Brazil Chile Czech Republic France Greece Guatemala Hungary
Italy Japan Poland Portugal Singapore South Korea Switzerland
Thailand Turkey Ukraine Vietnam

Oxford is a registered trade mark of Oxford University Press in the UK and in certain
other countries.

Published in the United States by Oxford University Press Inc., New York

First published 2008

Edited and designed by The Open University.

Typeset by SR Nova Pvt. Ltd, Bangalore, India.

Printed and bound in the United Kingdom by Latimer Trend & Company Ltd, Plymouth.

This book forms part of the Open University course SDK125 *Introducing Health Sciences: A Case
Study Approach*. Details of this and other Open University courses can be obtained from the Student
Registration and Enquiry Service, The Open University, PO Box 197, Milton Keynes MK7 6BJ,
United Kingdom:
tel. +44 (0)870 333 4340, email general-enquiries@open.ac.uk.

http://www.open.ac.uk

British Library Cataloguing in Publication Data available on request

Library of Congress Cataloging in Publication Data available on request

ISBN 9780 1992 3731 9

10 9 8 7 6 5 4 3 2 1

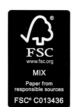

The paper used in this
publication contains pulp
sourced from forests
independently certified to the
Forest Stewardship Council
(FSC) principles and criteria.
Chain of custody certification
allows the pulp from these
forests to be tracked to the end
use (see www.fsc.org).

ABOUT THIS BOOK

This book and the accompanying material on DVD present the final case study in a series of seven, under the collective title *Introducing Health Sciences: A Case Study Approach*. Together they form an Open University (OU) course for students beginning the first year of an undergraduate programme in Health Sciences. Each case study has also been designed to 'stand alone' for readers studying it in isolation from the rest of the course, either as part of an educational programme at another institution, or for general interest and self-directed study.

Visual Impairment is a multidisciplinary introduction to eye defects and diseases that affect millions of people worldwide, and explains how many of these defects and diseases can be overcome or ameliorated by relatively inexpensive technologies. We have included aspects of the biology, physics, chemistry and epidemiology of the topic, and discuss the impact of modern human living environments. No previous experience of studying science has been assumed and new concepts and specialist terminology are explained with examples and illustrations. There is some mathematical content associated with the physics of light, but it is fully explained in the text and in worked examples on the DVD.

To help you plan your study of this material, there are a number of 'icons' in the margin to indicate different types of activity which have been included to help you develop and practise particular skills. This icon 💿 indicates when to undertake an activity on the accompanying DVD. You will need to 'run' the DVD programs on your computer because they are *interactive*, and this function doesn't operate on a domestic DVD-player. The DVD presents interactive activities: a video that gives an insight into the personal experience of blindness; two guided activities introducing the physics of the eye and the use of spectacles to correct certain types of poor sight; two activities showing the use of laser surgery and contact lenses, and a video showing how a variety of treatments can be brought to poor rural areas in developing countries although some sight-saving operations are too costly for the majority of the population.

Activities involving pencil-and-paper exercises are indicated by this icon 📝, and if you need a calculator you will see 🖩. Some additional activities for Open University students only are described in a *Companion* text, which is not available outside the OU course. These are indicated by this icon 📖 in the margin. References to activities for OU students are given in the margins of the book and should not interrupt your concentration if you are not studying it as part of an OU course.

At various points in the book, you will find 'boxed' material of two types: Explanation Boxes and Enrichment Boxes. The Explanation Boxes contain basic concepts explained in the kind of detail that someone who is completely new to the health sciences is likely to want. The Enrichment Boxes contain extension material, included for added interest, particularly if you already have some knowledge of basic science. If you are studying this book as part of an OU course, you should note that the Explanation Boxes contain material that is *essential* to your learning and which therefore may be *assessed*. However, the content of the Enrichment Boxes will *not* be tested in the course assessments.

The authors' intention is to bring you into the subject, develop confidence through activities and guidance, and provide a stepping stone into further study. The most important terms appear in **bold** font in the text at the point where they are first defined, and these terms are also in bold in the index at the end of the book. Understanding of the meaning and uses of the bold terms is essential (i.e. assessable) if you are an OU student.

Active engagement with the material throughout this book is encouraged by numerous 'in text' questions, indicated by a diamond symbol (◆), followed immediately by our suggested answers. It is good practice always to cover the answer and attempt your own response to the question before reading ours. At the end of each chapter, there is a summary of the key points and a list of the main learning outcomes, followed by self-assessment questions to enable you to test your own learning. The answers to these questions are at the back of the book.

Internet database (ROUTES)

A large amount of valuable information is available via the internet. To help OU students and other readers of books in this series to access good quality sites without having to search for hours, the OU has developed a collection of internet resources on a searchable database called ROUTES. All websites included in the database are selected by academic staff or subject-specialist librarians. The content of each website is evaluated to ensure that it is accurate, well presented and regularly updated. A description is included for each of the resources.

The website address for ROUTES is: http://routes.open.ac.uk/

Entering the Open University course code 'SDK125' in the search box will retrieve all the resources that have been recommended for this book. Alternatively, if you want to search for any resources on a particular subject, type in the words which best describe the subject you are interested in (for example, 'contact lenses'), or browse the alphabetical list of subjects.

Authors' acknowledgements

As ever in The Open University, this book and DVD combine the efforts of many people with specialist skills and knowledge in different disciplines. The principal authors were Heather McLannahan and Hilary MacQueen (biology), Jamie Harle (physics), Lesley Smart (chemistry), Jeanne Katz (health and social care) and Basiro Davey (pubic health). Our contributions have been shaped and immeasurably enriched by the OU course team who helped us to plan the content and made numerous comments and suggestions for improvements as the material progressed through several drafts. It would be impossible to thank everyone personally, but we would like to acknowledge the help and support of academic colleagues who have contributed to this book (in alphabetical order of discipline): Carol Midgley and James Phillips (biology), Elizabeth Parvin (physics), Frederick Toates (psychology) and Kevin McConway (statistics). The media developers who contributed directly to the production of the audiovisual and multimedia components of the DVD were Steve Best, Greg Black, Owen Horn, Jo Mack and Brian Richardson.

We would also like to thank Professor Gary Rubin (Professor of Visual Rehabilitation), University College London for critical reading of the manuscript and helpful comments and our External Assessor, Professor Susan Standring (Head of Department of Anatomy and Human Sciences), Kings College London, whose detailed comments have contributed to the structure and content of the book and kept the needs of our intended readership to the fore.

Special thanks are due to all those involved in the OU production process, chief among them Joy Wilson and Dawn Partner, our wonderful Course Manager and Course Team Assistant, whose commitment, efficiency and unflagging good humour were at the heart of the endeavour. We also warmly acknowledge the contributions of our editor, Bina Sharma, whose skill has improved every aspect of this book; Steve Best, our graphic artist, who developed and drew all the diagrams; Sarah Hofton and Chris Hough, our graphic designers, who devised the page designs and layouts; and Martin Keeling, who carried out picture research and rights clearance. The media project managers were Judith Pickering and James Davies.

For the copublication process, we would especially like to thank Jonathan Crowe of Oxford University Press and, from within The Open University, Christianne Bailey (Media Developer, Copublishing). As is the custom, any small errors or shortcomings that have slipped in (despite our collective best efforts) remain the responsibility of the authors. We would be pleased to receive feedback on the book (favourable or otherwise). Please write to the address below.

Dr Basiro Davey, SDK125 Course Team Chair

Department of Life Sciences
The Open University
Walton Hall
Milton Keynes
MK7 6AA
United Kingdom

Environmental statement

Paper and board used in this publication is FSC certified.

Forestry Stewardship Council (FSC) is an independent certification, which certifies that the virgin pulp used to make the paper/board comes from traceable and sustainable sources from well-managed forests.

CONTENTS

The DVD activities associated with this book were written, designed and developed by Steve Best, Greg Black, Basiro Davey, Jamie Harle, Owen Horn, Jeanne Katz, Jo Mack, Heather McLannahan, Hilary MacQueen, Brian Richardson and Lesley Smart.

CHAPTER 1

A GLOBAL VIEW

1.1 The range of sight problems

This case study is about impaired sight and the many ways in which it can be improved, so the tone of this book is, we hope, optimistic. In our daily lives, we rely on all of our senses in order to interact with other people and the world around us. But sight is deemed the most important sense according to a survey of adults in the United Kingdom (UK) by the Royal National Institute of Blind People (RNIB), which found that 90% most feared losing their sight (McLaughlan, 2006).

◆ Suggest some reasons why sight holds such an important place in our lives.

◆ It affects most aspects of daily functioning, including the ability to care for ourselves and others, move from place to place, participate in education, make a living and enjoy social interactions and leisure activities such as reading and watching television. People who lose their sight also lose some aspects of the independence they experienced in their sighted lives.

Like 'hard of hearing' which doesn't assume someone is profoundly deaf, **visual impairment** refers to a range of conditions, from total loss of sight (blindness), to partial sight loss. The current definition in the *International Statistical Classification of Diseases and Related Health Problems* (ICD10) excludes vision loss that could be corrected by spectacles, but includes vision loss that could be corrected by surgery. There are therefore a great many people who we might think of as being visually impaired because, for the lack of a pair of spectacles, they cannot see clearly. However, this group of people are not counted in official statistics on the extent of visual impairment.

Spectacles are also known as 'glasses' in the UK.

This means that the data collected by the World Health Organization (WHO) on visual impairment give a considerable underestimation of the number of people who have a **visual disability**, i.e. an impairment that interferes with the normal day-to-day functions of the affected person. Globally, over 2 billion people, or one-third of the world's population, would have a visual disability were it not for corrective treatments such as spectacles (Sachdev, 2005).

In this case study, the data related to visual impairment have been assembled using the narrower definition given above. However, in the 21st century there is much discussion about the need to redefine the term to include people whose visual loss could be corrected if they wore spectacles. There are places in the case study where, for practical reasons, this wider definition of visual impairment is used.

The range of effects of visual impairments is very varied: for some people the view of distant objects is blurred, whereas others cannot see close objects clearly, or they see only a partial view of the scene around them. Later in the case study, you will learn the technical definitions of important terms involved in classifying visual impairments, but functional descriptions are adequate at this stage.

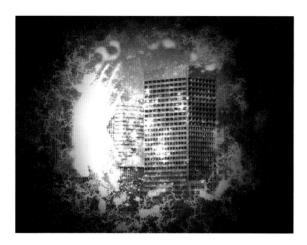

Figure 1.1 Office blocks as seen by someone with poor peripheral vision, sometimes called tunnel vision. (Source: Phototake Inc./ Photolibrary)

Visual acuity refers to your ability to see detail. *Visual field* refers to the entire extent of what you can see while looking straight ahead, so it includes your peripheral vision. People whose peripheral vision is curtailed see the world as though from inside a tunnel (Figure 1.1); other people may only have peripheral vision and be unable to see objects straight in front of them.

In Chapter 2, we explain how the structures of the eye and their connections to the brain produce the perception of sight, and how the physical properties of light are relevant to an understanding of vision. Most people see a wide range of colours, but a minority (mainly male) have impaired colour vision, as you will learn in Chapter 3. Spectacles are prescribed to correct 'short' and 'long' sight, the so-called *refractive errors* – a term explained in Chapter 4 with the help of a DVD activity on how spectacles work. Chapter 5 reveals how contact lenses and laser surgery can correct certain visual impairments, and Chapter 6 describes the **chronic conditions** responsible for the majority of blindness and partial sight globally. Chronic conditions (wherever they occur in the body) are characterised by their gradual onset and inexorable progression, which can result in irreversible damage.

'Vision 2020: the Right to Sight', a joint programme of intervention by WHO and the International Agency for the Prevention of Blindness (IAPB), aims to eliminate avoidable blindness worldwide by 2020. Box 1.1 introduces the six most common **priority eye diseases** targeted by this campaign.

Box 1.1 (Explanation) The six most common 'priority eye diseases' (WHO, 2007a)

These brief descriptions include some terms explained fully in later chapters.

Refractive errors and low vision. Refractive errors occur when the eye cannot focus correctly, and include *myopia* (my-oh-pee-ah; short-sightedness), and *hyperopia* (high-per-oh-pee-ah; long-sightedness), with or without astigmatism (as-tig-mat-izm; a defect that results in distorted images). Chapter 4 explains refractive errors and low vision in more detail.

Cataract is clouding of the lens of the eye, which impedes the passage of light. Most cases of cataract are a result of the ageing process, but occasionally children can be born with the condition, or a cataract may develop after an eye injury or inflammation (Figure 1.2).

Glaucoma is a group of diseases involving damage to the optic nerves that take signals from the eyes to the brain; it is most commonly due to a build-up of pressure within the eyeball.

Age-related macular degeneration (AMD) involves loss of vision in the centre of the visual field; it may involve a reduction in blood flow to the

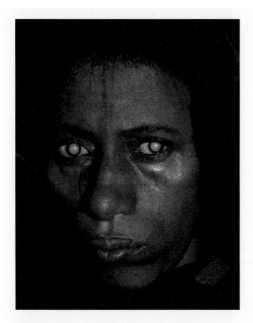

Figure 1.2 Woman with bilateral cataracts. (Source: WHO/Serge Resnikoff)

macula, the central area of the retina (a structure at the back of the eye, described in Chapter 2).

Diabetic retinopathy can occur in people who have had *diabetes mellitus* for several years. The retina is damaged as a result of changes in the blood vessels supplying it, including the excessive growth of new blood vessels.

Trachoma is caused by a microbe (*Chlamydia trachomatis*; clam-id-ee-ah track-oh-matis) spread through contact with the pus discharged from infected eyes (e.g. on fingers) and through transmission by eye-seeking flies. After years of repeated infection, the inside of the eyelid may be scarred so severely that the eyelid turns inward and the lashes rub on the eyeball, scarring the cornea (the front of the eye), leading to irreversible damage and blindness.

Diabetes mellitus is a condition in which lack of the hormone insulin, or insensitivity to insulin, results in poor control of blood sugar levels; if untreated, this can damage blood vessels over time.

1.2 How many people have impaired sight?

Total blindness, the complete absence of any visual perception, is relatively rare. The statistics quoted in this section use an internationally accepted definition of blindness in which some detection of light, shape or colour may be possible. (The definition is based on measurements of visual acuity in the better eye and is sometimes called 'legal blindness' because it qualifies the person for certain benefits or services.)

A major WHO survey estimated that in 2002 a total of 0.6% of the world's population were blind – which may sound a small proportion, but it represents 37 million people (Resnikoff et al., 2004). The same survey estimated that 161 million people were visually impaired. Some later estimates have suggested that the total number with visual disabilities is 314 million, or about 5% of the world's population; this included 153 million people who would not have been visually disabled if spectacles could have been provided (WHO, 2006).

Like all diseases and disorders, visual impairment is not distributed equally between different populations. The WHO divides the world into six regions for the purposes of data collection; although some regions include both 'developed' and 'developing' countries (e.g. 'The Americas' includes countries as diverse as the USA and Nicaragua), some idea of the extent to which disadvantage and visual impairment are linked can be gained from Table 1.1 overleaf.

Definitions of 'developed' and 'developing' countries include national income and indicators such as literacy rates and access to clean water, sanitation and healthcare.

Table 1.1 Global estimates of blindness and visual impairment in 2002 by WHO region (in millions and as a percentage of the total). (Sources: Resnikoff et al., 2004)

WHO region	Africa	The Americas	Eastern Mediterranean region	Europe	South East Asian region	Western Pacific region	Total
population (millions)	672.2	852.6	502.8	877.9	1590.8	1717.5	6213.9
% of global population	11%	14%	8%	14%	25.5%	27.5%	100%
number of blind people (millions)	6.8	2.4	4.0	2.7	11.6	9.3	36.9
% of global total of blind people	18%	7%	11%	7%	32%	25%	100%
number with visual impairment (millions)	26.8	15.5	16.5	15.5	45.1	41.8	161.2
% of global total of visually impaired people	17%	10%	10%	10%	27%	26%	100%

◆ What do you notice when you compare the data for Africa and Europe?

◆ 11% of the global population live in Africa, but it has 18% of the world's blind people and 17% of the global burden of visual impairment. Conversely, the proportion of blind people in Europe is 7% of the global total and the global burden of visual impairment is 10% – well below the European 'share' of the world's population (14%).

1.2.1 The influence of location, age and gender

Blindness and visual impairment have far reaching social, economic and developmental implications. They are a harbinger of poverty. In fact, they perpetuate it. Moreover, there is increasing evidence that women suffer a disproportionately higher burden of visual disability.

(Dr Gro Harlem Brundtland, former WHO Director General, in a speech on World Blindness Day, 2002)

Developing countries often have a disproportionate level of blindness and visual impairment compared with developed countries.

◆ Can you suggest some explanations?

◆ The most obvious is lack of services to treat correctable sight loss, and the difficulties due to cost or distance that many people face in accessing whatever treatment is available. Some infectious eye diseases (e.g. trachoma, Box 1.1) are more likely to occur in tropical conditions, or where there is poor access to clean water and sanitation. Lifelong exposure to 'blinding' sunshine damages the eyes, and there are more injuries where eye protection (e.g. goggles) is rarely used in occupations that pose a significant risk (Figure 1.3).

In all countries, the risk factor most strongly associated with visual impairment is age: for example, over 80% of all blind people are aged 50 years or more. Chronic eye diseases take time to develop and some deterioration in vision is a normal part of ageing. Age-related cataract is the major cause of global blindness, accounting for 48% of all cases in 2002 (Resnikoff et al., 2004).

Gender is another important dimension: for every man with a visual impairment, between 1.5 and 2.2 women are affected, even after adjusting for the fact that women on average tend to live longer than men.

◆ Why is it important to make this adjustment for age?

◆ Since visual impairments become more common with age, unless this is taken into account, it might simply be that more women are affected because the female population contains a larger proportion of older individuals.

Women in disadvantaged circumstances experience a higher burden of visual impairment partly because some aspects of their lives place them at increased risk of developing eye diseases or sight loss. For example, women in many rural populations in developing countries are persistently exposed to smoke from indoor cooking fires and this places them at increased risk of developing cataracts. Some women and girls may have a significantly worse diet than men throughout life, and vitamin A deficiency can cause a variety of eye problems, including blindness (Chapter 3). But the major factor is that women are more likely to be denied adequate treatment for visual impairments, which in many societies is preferentially offered to men because of social, cultural or religious reasons (Gooding, 2006).

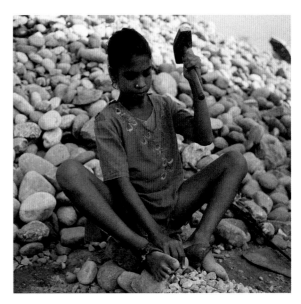

Figure 1.3 A young Bangladeshi girl chipping stones for road building is at high risk of an eye injury. (Source: Shezad Noohrani/Still Pictures)

Indoor smoke is also a factor in the development of chronic obstructive pulmonary disease (COPD) – the subject of another book in this series, *Chronic Obstructive Pulmonary Disease: A Forgotten Killer* (Midgley, 2008).

1.3 Living with visual impairment

1.3.1 Impact of visual impairment on children

In 2002, there were around 1.4 million blind children. Human babies are taught a great deal about the world and how to interact with it by watching their carers; for example, they learn how to hold a spoon the right way up to feed efficiently. Parenting a blind child requires more time and planning and is also more expensive, because special equipment and a constant carer may be needed to support the child's development and ensure their safety. Not being able to see, and thus mimic behaviour, can mean that the child does not learn social behaviour in conventional ways and cannot understand non-verbal cues. As they grow up, this makes it more difficult to prepare for independent living.

Educating children with visual impairments in high-income countries has been improved in recent years by advances in computer-aided technologies and optical and audio aids, but services even in a relatively wealthy country such as the UK fall short of those needed. However, three-quarters of blind children live in developing countries, where the *prevalence rate* (the total number of blind children, expressed as a rate per 1000 children) may be as high as 1.5 per 1000, compared with around 0.3 per 1000 in the developed world. State aid is rarely available in developing countries and the care and education of blind children places a huge burden on their family or community and most miss out on education altogether. Life expectancy is also reduced: up to 60% of children in the poorest countries die within a year of becoming blind, either from the disease that has caused the blindness, or as a consequence of the disadvantages conferred by being blind (Gilbert and Foster, 2001).

For every blind child there are many more with uncorrected visual disabilities. Husan's story (Vignette 1.1) illustrates some of the difficulties they face.

Vignette 1.1   Husan's story

Traumatic injuries are a common cause of eye damage in children. Husan Dad Shah from Pakistan was 12 when he ruptured an eye while playing with a stick. An initial operation was unsuccessful in restoring his sight and the eye later developed a cataract. Husan explained: 'My eye was looking ugly and this worsened my confidence. I was not sure that I would be able to see this world again with both my eyes. I left my studies and considered myself useless'. He was nervous about seeking further treatment, but when he was 13 his family persuaded him to travel to a Sightsavers clinic in Karachi, where he underwent eye surgery which restored his sight and improved the appearance of his eye (Figure 1.4). 'Seeing the world again with both eyes makes me feel happy, confident and courageous towards life. I am interested to go back to my village and start my studies again… This seems essential to me to carry out some good works for others.'

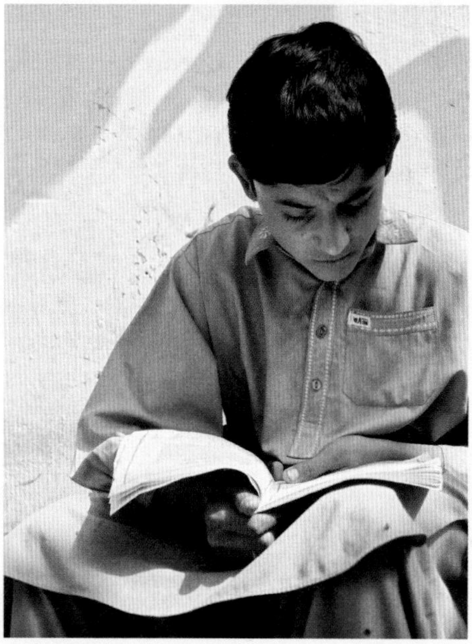

Figure 1.4   Husan can read again. (Source: Jamshyd Masud/Sightsavers International)

Sightsavers International is a charity that works to combat blindness in some of the world's poorest countries, restoring sight through specialist treatment and eye care and providing support to people who are irreversibly blind.

1.3.2   Impact of visual impairment in adults

Although the onset of sight loss in later life may be gradual, it is not always possible to put strategies into place that will allow the individual to continue living independently and earn a living or access education (Figure 1.5). In agricultural communities, someone who can no longer see small objects clearly at close range may be unable to plant seeds or weed crops. As sight deteriorates, the jobs that can be done become less skilled and the individual may lose their income and status within their community. Women may become marginalised if they can no longer manage the domestic tasks they have traditionally fulfilled. The prognosis for blind people living in developing countries is poor; on average they die within four years of losing their sight (The Fred Hollows Foundation, 2007).

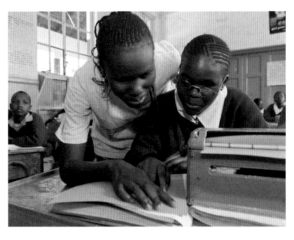

Figure 1.5   Angeline Akai is a totally blind teacher who lives in the Kibera shantytown in Nairobi, Kenya. She has found it hard to get work in competition with sighted colleagues for scarce teaching jobs. (Source: Georgina Cranston/Sightsavers International)

The outlook can also be serious in developed countries. Canadian research showed that people with irreversible visual loss are twice as likely to fall, four times as likely to fracture a hip, three times as likely to suffer clinical depression and twice as likely to die as those of similar age with good sight (CNIB symposium, 2004).

However, with determination and adequate support, blind and partially sighted people can lead productive and interesting lives, as Activity 1.1 demonstrates.

Activity 1.1   Adjusting to sight loss

Allow 30 minutes

Now is the ideal time to study the video 'Adjusting to sight loss' on the DVD associated with this book. Derek Child, Head of Equality and Diversity at the Open University in the UK, describes some aspects of his daily life since he became totally blind at the age of 29. Take particular note of what he says on the following topics:

(a)   What difficulties does Derek refer to in getting safely from place to place, and how has a guide dog increased his independence (Figure 1.6)?

(b)   How has Braille, the touch language developed for blind people (Box 1.2 overleaf), and modern computer-aided technologies enabled him to maintain a demanding career?

(c)   What reasons does he give for the inequalities that exist in services and support for blind and partially sighted people even in relatively wealthy countries such as the UK?

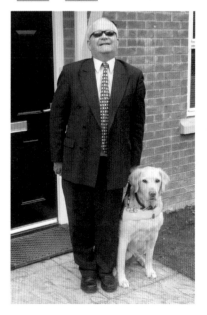

Figure 1.6   Derek Child and his guide dog Baxter. (Source: Derek Child)

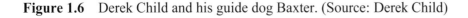

Box 1.2 (Enrichment) Braille

The Frenchman Louis Braille (1809–1852) was accidentally blinded when he was three. In his teens, he started to develop the system of writing named after him, in which each letter of the alphabet is represented by dots in six positions, arranged in two columns of three dots each (Figure 1.7).

In basic Braille there are 64 combinations (including one in which no dots are raised); more advanced Braille systems use dots to represent combinations of letters. Courses to learn how to read it typically take 18–24 months. (Derek, in Activity 1.1, taught himself to read Braille.)

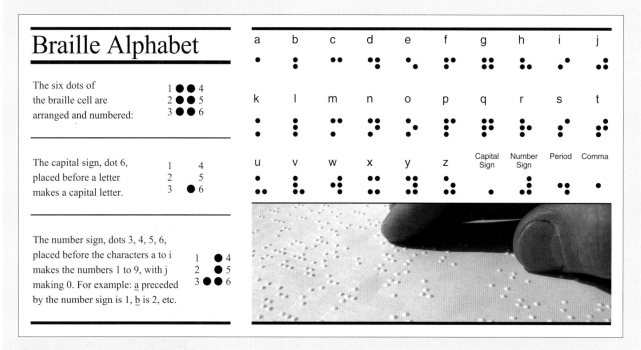

Figure 1.7 The Braille Alphabet card and (inset) using Braille: notice that the dots are raised from the page. (Source: Tim Pohl/istockphoto).

According to the RNIB, aids such as large-print books, 'talking books' on audiotape and audio-descriptions of television programmes are in limited supply and should be much more widely available if visually impaired people are to enter fully into the normal daily life of their society. Studies undertaken by the RNIB (2005) have highlighted some of these difficulties; for example, although 94% of blind and partially sighted people watch television, 70% of this group experience difficulties in understanding what is going on.

1.3.3 Poverty and visual impairment

In addition to the estimated 37 million blind and 161 million visually impaired people, it is believed that a further 153 million people worldwide in 2002 were visually disabled because they were not provided with spectacles (WHO, 2006). Although most of the unmet need is in developing countries, studies of older people in developed countries have demonstrated that they often don't receive, or may not seek access to, services to treat visual disability. Lack of access is more apparent among older people with lower educational attainment and poor financial status (Jacobs et al., 2005). Another revealing example is that African Americans, who are at greater risk of age-related visual impairment than their white counterparts, are less likely to have seen an eye specialist (Orr et al., 1999).

◆ Can you suggest what underlies these inequalities?

◆ Disadvantage lies at the heart of the problem. People on low incomes (especially in a fee-paying healthcare system such as that in the USA) may not be able to afford eye-care services, or even the transport costs to reach them. Where educational attainment is low, people are less likely to know what services exist or how to obtain them. Reticence about seeking help may also be a feature of some people's attitudes.

The relationship between disability and poverty works in both directions: just as the poor are most at risk of suffering a visual impairment, so too the disabilities resulting from it promote or exacerbate poverty (Gooding, 2006). For example, unemployment is high among people with visual impairments (particularly women). If sight can be improved enough for the person to return to work, the life chances of an entire household may be increased.

Finally, it is worth drawing attention to the huge financial implications of visual impairment for nations as well as individuals. Vision 2020 estimates the global cost of lost productivity due to uncorrected visual impairment is US$42 billion per year. If the campaign succeeds in eliminating avoidable or treatable visual impairments by 2020, the economic gain would be US$102 billion (Frick and Foster, 2003).

Summary of Chapter 1

1.1 Visual impairment ranges from a total absence of sight to partial sight loss that cannot be further improved by surgical procedures or wearing spectacles. Visual disability refers to reduced functionality as a result of sight loss.

1.2 Two billion people wear spectacles and would be visually disabled without them; a further 153 million need but do not have spectacles to correct their sight.

1.3 About 5% of the world's population suffer from visual disabilities and 0.6% are blind; the majority live in developing countries and women are disproportionately represented.

1.4 Vision 2020 aims to eliminate avoidable blindness by targeting priority eye diseases, including refractive errors and low vision, cataracts, glaucoma, age-related macular degeneration (AMD), diabetic retinopathy and trachoma.

1.5 Access to services to treat visual impairment, provide spectacles and other aids and to support blind and partially sighted people is unequally distributed between and within countries, along lines of poverty and disadvantage.

1.6   Visual impairment and visual disabilities are major causes of poverty, lack of education, unemployment and loss of status, especially (but not exclusively) in developing countries.

1.7   The independence and productivity of blind and partially sighted people can be greatly enhanced by computer-aided technologies and other enabling services.

Learning outcomes for Chapter 1

After studying this chapter and its associated activities, you should be able to:

LO 1.1   Define and use in context, or recognise definitions and applications of, each of the terms printed in **bold** in the text. (Question 1.1)

LO 1.2   Summarise the main patterns in the distribution of visual impairment in different parts of the world and in different age-groups, genders and social circumstances, and suggest reasons why some groups in a population are at greater risk. (Questions 1.1 and 1.3)

LO 1.3   Illustrate the consequences of sight loss for practical, personal and social functioning in children and adults, and identify some ways in which disability resulting from visual impairment may be alleviated. (Questions 1.2 and 1.3 and DVD Activity 1.1)

Self-assessment questions for Chapter 1

Question 1.1 (LOs 1.1 and 1.2)

In 2002, cataracts accounted for 48% of all cases of blindness worldwide. What is a cataract and which age-groups are most at risk?

Question 1.2 (LO 1.3)

What are the four ways in which Derek Child (DVD Activity 1.1) claims that blind and partially sighted people in developed countries are disadvantaged in terms of the services they need?

Question 1.3 (LOs 1.2 and 1.3)

What is meant by the claim that visual impairment and poverty interact in a 'vicious cycle of disadvantage'?

CHAPTER 2

HOW THE EYE WORKS

2.1 Eye structure and function

Having established that poor sight is a problem for a great many people, we now turn our attention to the organ that collects visual information – the eye. Knowledge of the eye's structure and the way that it functions enables many causes of visual impairment to be understood. As a result, corrective strategies can be developed to improve or restore sight.

The human eye is a ball-like structure roughly spherical in shape, but it has a bulge at the front. This bulging area is the part of the eye that we can see when we look at someone's face. Most of the eyeball fits into a bony socket in the skull known as the orbital cavity (Figure 2.1a). A hammock of fatty tissue cushions the eyeball so that it lodges snugly into the orbital cavity.

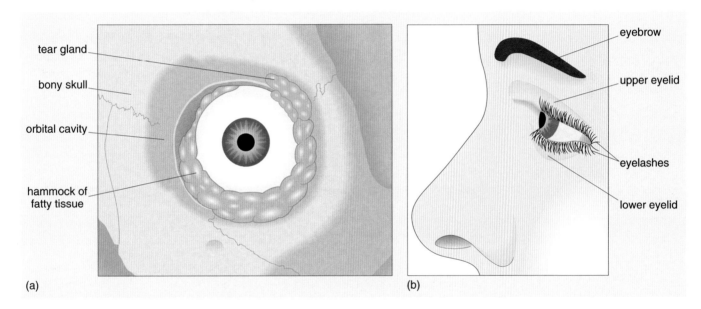

(a)   (b)

Figure 2.1 Diagram of the eye showing protective structures around it. (a) View from the front with skin removed. (b) Side view.

◆ Eyes are delicate and need protection. In Figure 2.1, which structures appear to protect them?

◆ The bony skull and the fatty tissue protect much of the eye. The eyelids close over the front of the eye to provide additional protection.

You might also have suggested that the eyelashes would offer some protection, as indeed they do. Along with the eyebrows they keep a certain amount of dust and sweat from falling into the eye. Figure 2.1a also shows the tear gland. Tears have an important protective role. Fluid secreted from the tear gland spreads across the front surface of the eye and drains away from the eye into the nasal cavity, the air-filled space behind the nose. This is why your nose runs when your eyes water. Tears lubricate the front of the eyeball as well as the inside of the eyelid, ensuring that the delicate tissues covering these surfaces, known as the conjunctiva (kon-junk-tye-vah), do not dry out. To maintain complete coverage of tear fluid over the eye, the eyelids briefly close about once every four seconds in the reflex action of blinking.

Tears also help to wash away dust and debris and provide nutrients such as glucose to the tissues at the front of the eye. If you have ever licked away tears you may have thought that they were no more than salty water but in fact they also contain:

- lipids (oily secretions that assist with the prevention of dehydration)
- antibodies (specialised proteins that are secreted by **cells** of the *immune system* which defends the body against pathogens and other 'non-self' particles such as pollen)
- lysozyme (a bactericidal enzyme, i.e. a protein that specifically aids in the destruction of bacteria).

◈ Give some instances of occasions when tears are produced particularly copiously, i.e. your eyes 'water'.

◆ Your eyes 'water' or 'weep':

- when exposed to certain chemicals, e.g. smoke or onion fumes
- when you have a speck of dirt in your eye
- if you suffer from hay fever
- as a result of strong emotion.

◈ In which of the situations above might tears provide protection?

◆ Tears can help to wash out dirt, smoke and other chemicals and particles such as pollen.

Unfortunately the immune system of people with hay fever reacts to 'non-self' proteins such as pollen proteins (that are tolerated by other people) by mounting an *inflammatory response* resulting in symptoms like a runny nose and watering eyes. So even here tears provide a protective response, albeit a misplaced one.

Emotion is a bit more of a puzzle, but tears that are produced under stressful or emotional circumstances have been found to contain many toxic biological substances. So, tears have been proposed as a means of removing these chemicals that are produced by the body during times of emotional stress!

By just looking into someone's eyes, you would have no idea that the eye was a ball-like structure. What you see is almond-shaped, fringed by eyelids and lashes (Figure 2.2). At the centre is a black disc, the **pupil**. This is, literally, a hole through which light enters the eye. The pupil is surrounded by a solid structure, the **iris**, which has the appearance of a coloured disc (or more correctly a ring, or annulus, because of the hole – the pupil – at its centre). The iris is made of smooth muscle tissue and has pigment cells that bestow the characteristic colour. Contraction and relaxation of the iris muscles alters the size of the pupil, thereby regulating the amount of light that enters the eye.

A reflex is an automatic response to a stimulus. It cannot be controlled by will-power.

Cells are the smallest individual units of an organism. Pathogens are harmful microbes such as bacteria, viruses or fungi that cause disease.

The process of inflammation is discussed in another book in this series (Midgley, 2008).

There are three types of muscle in the body: skeletal muscles, which move bones; cardiac muscle, found in the heart; and smooth muscle, which contracts and relaxes without conscious control.

The 'white of the eye' is called the sclera (skle-rah), a tough tissue that envelopes the whole of the eyeball to maintain its shape. You can see in Figure 2.3 that the sclera is continuous with the **cornea** (corn-ee-ah). The cornea differs most obviously from the sclera in that it is transparent. A transparent substance is one that allows light to pass through it unaltered. This means that you cannot see it (in the same way that you cannot 'see' clean glass). Transparent tissues are needed at the front of the eye in the same manner that transparent glass is needed to illuminate a room during daytime.

The bulk of the cornea tissue is called **stroma**, which is formed from long thin fibres of the protein collagen aligned in such a way that light can pass through unaltered. The cornea also serves as a tough outer surface, like the skin, and has **epithelial cells** (ep-ee-thee-lee-al) at the surface. Epithelial cells form a protective barrier and are found on the outer surface of many body tissues. Corneal epithelial cells are continuously worn away because of eyeball motion and blinking, so they require constant replacement.

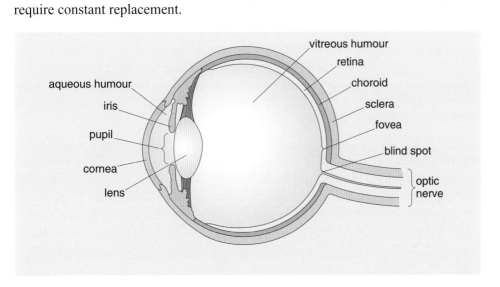

Figure 2.2   The eye viewed from the front.

Figure 2.3   Cross-section of the human eye. The terms fovea and blind spot will be explained later.

The cornea lies in front of the iris, separated from it by a transparent fluid called **aqueous** (ay-kwee-us) **humour**. Notice also the **vitreous** (vit-ree-us) **humour**, a gelatinous fluid with a thick consistency within the eyeball that helps maintain eyeball shape. It, too, is transparent.

There is another transparent structure, the **lens**, lying behind the iris, but you cannot see this through the pupil when you gaze into someone's eyes. Nor do you see the back of the eye; in fact, you do not see anything, just blackness. The reason for this is that light passes into the eye through several transparent layers but is then captured inside the eye. This light then falls on the **retina**, the innermost layer of the wall of the eye and the layer that contains visual receptor cells. These are the cells of the eye that are sensitive to light. Chapter 3 examines in detail the interaction of light with these receptor cells which forms the

Aqueous describes the physical state in which a substance is dissolved in water.

biological basis of sight. Any light that penetrates through the retina is captured very effectively by the next layer of the eye, the **choroid** (cor-oid).

To understand how the eye processes light entering through the iris, it is first necessary to think about what light is and how its properties enable the sense of vision.

2.2 Light

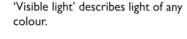

'Visible light' describes light of any colour.

Light (or in scientific terms, *visible light*) is a form of energy that travels from one place to another at very high speed. Because light travels so quickly, the information it transfers from the surroundings is up to date. Furthermore as light travels in straight lines through air, one can reliably trace its origin. Therefore it is an excellent means of carrying information about your local environment. Light can travel through many different substances or **media** (singular: medium).

◈ Suggest some media through which light can travel.

◆ Common examples include air, water and glass.

These media all have the property of being transparent (or near transparent). Light (or some light) can penetrate through, so that the eye can collect visual information about objects that lie within or beyond these media. The process where light passes through a substance is known as **transmission**. However, not all media transmit light; some can stop light, a process known as **absorption**. Drawing the curtains in a room is a simple way of turning a window frame and fittings from a structure that *transmits* light into one that stops light passing through – i.e. *absorbs* light.

The thin layer of light-absorbing material in a curtain contrasts greatly with the many kilometres of air that light from the Sun is able to travel through to reach the surface of the Earth. This shows how different media have vastly different light absorption and transmission characteristics. The cornea and lens, at the front of the eye, must be transparent to allow good transmission of light into the eye. But this can change with the development of a cataract, where the lens of the eye loses some transmission ability and instead absorbs some of the incoming light. (Chapter 6 looks at cataracts and other visual impairments.)

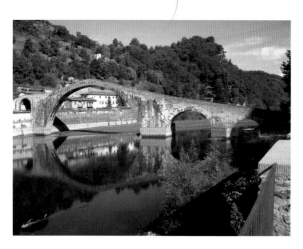

Figure 2.4 The Devil's Bridge in Tuscany, Italy. (Source: Lesley Smart)

Light can also be reflected. **Reflection** occurs at the junction or *interface* of two media, with light being returned in a predictable direction within the first medium. Look at Figure 2.4, which is a photograph of a famous bridge in Tuscany, Italy. Studying this photograph, you will notice that there is a 'copy' of the bridge visible upon the water's surface. This copy is inverted, or upside-down.

Reflection can be explained by thinking about how the bridge and its inverted 'copy' appear in the photograph. The bridge is apparent because light travels directly from the bridge to the camera through the air. The *inverted* bridge is apparent because light travels from the bridge to the water, and is then reflected in a new direction that takes it to the camera. The air–water interface reflects light from the bridge, and the result is that the inverted bridge appears to come from the points of reflection on the water's surface.

Up to now we have not addressed what light is, and this is an essential part of explaining the detection of light by the retina at the back of the eye. Light is a form of **electromagnetic radiation**. This is a type of energy that can be described both as a wave, and as a flow of 'packets' of energy, as will be explained later on. Electromagnetic radiation can travel through many media, and indeed through a **vacuum**, which is a volume in which no atoms or molecules are present and therefore has zero pressure (such as is found in space).

While you may not have come across the term electromagnetic radiation, you are no doubt familiar with several forms of it. The full **spectrum**, or range of frequencies, of electromagnetic radiation is shown in Figure 2.5. It can be seen that visible light makes up only a very small region of this spectrum. Other regions include radio waves (used to transmit radio and television signals) and X-rays (used in hospitals for medical purposes). There are a variety of technological applications for different regions of the electromagnetic spectrum. This is because different regions exhibit different characteristics; for example, transmission and absorption vary greatly. A battery-operated two-way radio can carry voice messages over several kilometres using radio waves, while a similarly powered TV remote control, which uses infrared radiation, can barely transmit across the length of a room.

Atoms are the smallest particles of a particular element (there are 92 naturally occurring elements, e.g. oxygen, hydrogen). Molecules are made from two or more atoms bonded together (e.g. an oxygen atom and two hydrogen atoms bond together to form a water molecule).

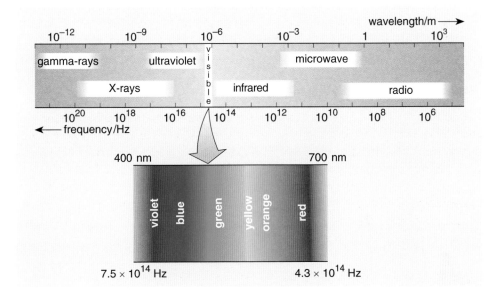

Figure 2.5   The electromagnetic spectrum. Note that the frequencies in this spectrum are expressed as 'powers of ten' where, for example, the frequency of a microwave can be 10^{10} Hz. 10^{10} (spoken as 'ten to the ten') is a scientific way of writing ten billion (i.e. 1 with 10 noughts). The unit Hz will be explained later.

Electromagnetic radiation is often explained as a **wave**. A wave is a constantly repeating variation that transfers energy from one position to another. All waves can be described by their properties of wavelength, frequency and speed. An everyday example of a wave is a water wave, where water height at a 'snapshot' in time is shown in Figure 2.6 overleaf. The distance between one peak and the next is known as the **wavelength** (measured in metres with the symbol m). The number of times per second that this variation occurs at a stationary point (i.e. how often the peak of a wave rolls over you if you are standing in the sea) is known as the **frequency** of the wave (measured in cycles per second or s^{-1}).

$m\ s^{-1}$ is the scientific way of writing metres per second, sometimes written m/s. The superscript '-1' is used to indicate 'one over' or 'per', so s^{-1} is 'per second' and $m\ s^{-1}$ is 'metres per second'.

An equivalent and more convenient unit than cycles per second is the unit of hertz (her-ts, symbol Hz). The distance that the wave travels in one second is the speed of the wave (measured in metres per second or m s^{-1}). Now study Box 2.1.

Figure 2.6 A water wave observed at a particular time, showing variation of wave height with distance.

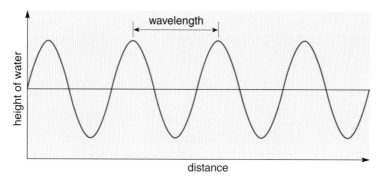

If you are not familiar with these terms, electric fields are the kind of field experienced during a thunder storm that leads to lightning strikes; magnetic fields are experienced in the vicinity of a magnet.

Box 2.1 (Explanation) **Electromagnetic waves**

Electromagnetic waves and water waves both involve a constantly repeating variation which leads to a transfer of energy. However, there are important differences between electromagnetic waves and water waves. A full description of electromagnetic waves needs more space and mathematics than we have here, but three key differences can be observed.

Firstly, water waves are due to a variation in one quantity with time (the height of water), while electromagnetic waves have variation in two quantities with time. These quantities are an electric field and a magnetic field. These fluctuate at a 'snapshot' in time in the synchronised manner shown in Figure 2.7; the electric field (blue) and magnetic field (orange) are always at right angles (90°) to each other and share a common frequency and wavelength that classifies the electromagnetic wave's region of the spectrum.

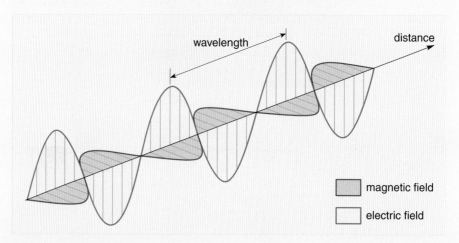

Figure 2.7 An electromagnetic wave, consisting of electric (blue) and magnetic (orange) fields that fluctuate as shown.

Water waves also require a medium for transmission (e.g. the sea). Electromagnetic waves can transmit even without a medium (i.e. in a vacuum). This property allows electromagnetic radiation from the Sun to reach the Earth through the vacuum of space.

And in addition, water waves and electromagnetic waves differ greatly from each other in terms of speed, frequency and wavelength. The speed of an electromagnetic wave in a vacuum is known as the 'speed of light' and has the approximate value of 3×10^8 m s^{-1} (the speed in air is only slightly less, but it is considerably reduced in some liquids or solids). In Section 2.3, you will compare values for water waves and the visible light region of the electromagnetic spectrum.

10^8 (said as 'ten to the eight') is a convenient way of writing 1 with eight noughts or 100 000 000.

◆ Looking back to Figure 2.5, between which regions of the electromagnetic spectrum does visible light fall?

◆ The infrared region (with a lower frequency) and the ultraviolet region (with a higher frequency).

The frequency range of the visible light region is very small, from a minimum of around 4.3×10^{14} Hz (lower than this is infrared) to a maximum of about 7.5×10^{14} Hz (higher than this is ultraviolet). The maximum frequency in the visible region is approximately double the minimum frequency. Looking at the adjacent infrared and ultraviolet regions, the maximum frequency of each region is approximately 100 times the value of the minimum frequency. So the eye can detect only a very small part of the electromagnetic spectrum, and this process will be explored in more detail in the next section.

Figure 2.5 shows that the maximum frequency of both infrared and ultraviolet regions is 100 times (10^2 times) the value of the minimum frequency.

2.3   Properties of light

Some of the properties of visible light can be investigated using glass prisms. These are thick triangular blocks of glass (Figure 2.8). When a beam of *white light* is passed through a prism, the light is seen to separate into a wide range of colours, arranged in the order of the rainbow, as shown. Furthermore, if a second prism is introduced, but inverted in relation to the first, then the separate colours can reform as a single beam of white light again (as shown in Figure 2.9 overleaf).

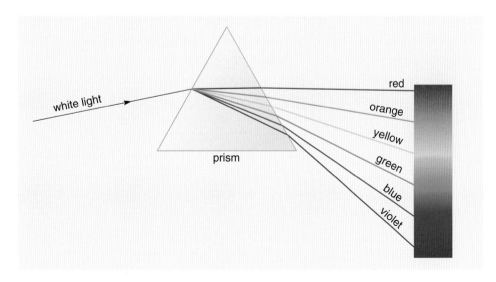

white light

prism

red
orange
yellow
green
blue
violet

Figure 2.8   White light is split into separate components by a prism. The components of light that we can see with the eye – from light with a red colour at one extreme to violet at the other – make up the visible region of the electromagnetic spectrum.

Figure 2.9 Passing white light through a prism shows that it consists of a mix of light waves, perceived by the eye as different colours. Each of the coloured rays shown here represents the path of a small spread of frequencies. Passing the spectrum of coloured rays through a second prism reconstitutes them into a single beam of white light.

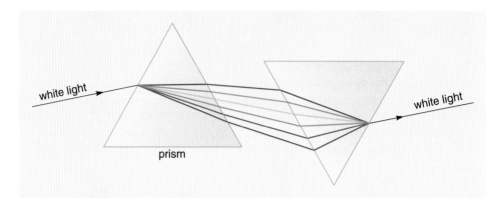

Equations are numbered so they can be referred back to later in the text.

These experiments show that white light is what the eye perceives when there is a simultaneous mix of light waves from all colours of the rainbow (i.e. the full range of frequencies within the visible light range of the electromagnetic spectrum).

The frequency and wavelength of a wave are related by its speed, expressed by the equation:

$$\text{speed} = \text{wavelength} \times \text{frequency}$$
$$(\text{m s}^{-1}) \qquad (\text{m}) \qquad (\text{s}^{-1} \text{ or Hz}) \tag{2.1}$$

Values of frequency (or wavelength) can be calculated for each colour of light, using the approximate value of the speed of light in air (3×10^8 m s^{-1}). However, the speed (in m s^{-1}) and frequency (in Hz) of light are very large numbers and the wavelength (in m) is a very small number, making calculations quite difficult.

An everyday example with more convenient values is a water wave, as shown earlier, in Figure 2.6.

Box 2.2 shows how Equation 2.1 can be used to determine properties of waves.

Box 2.2 (Explanation) **Rearranging equations**

The speed of a wave (in m s^{-1}) is related to its wavelength (in m) and frequency (in s^{-1} or Hz) by the following equation.

$$\text{speed} = \text{wavelength} \times \text{frequency} \tag{2.1}$$

This equation allows you to calculate the speed of the wave if both the wavelength and frequency are known. However, what if you want to calculate wavelength (or frequency) instead, using known values of the other terms?

This can be done by a process known as 'rearranging' the equation. First, you reverse the equation. Changing over the terms on each side of Equation 2.1 gives:

$$\text{wavelength} \times \text{frequency} = \text{speed} \tag{2.2}$$

Next, both sides of the equation are divided by frequency:

$$\frac{\text{wavelength} \times \text{frequency}}{\text{frequency}} = \frac{\text{speed}}{\text{frequency}} \qquad (2.3)$$

The left-hand side of Equation 2.3 now has frequency above and below the line, so they cancel each other out (because frequency divided by itself = 1). Cancelling the two frequency terms on the left-hand side gives the rearranged Equation 2.4 which enables you to calculate wavelength from speed and frequency:

$$\text{wavelength} = \frac{\text{speed}}{\text{frequency}} \qquad (2.4)$$

◆ Taking Equation 2.1, and working through the steps above, what equation can be written to calculate the frequency if you know the speed and wavelength? (Hint: again reverse the equation, but then divide by wavelength.)

◆ $\text{frequency} = \dfrac{\text{speed}}{\text{wavelength}}$ \qquad (2.5)

Equations 2.1, 2.4 and 2.5 can always be used to calculate the properties of waves, provided two of the three quantities (speed, wavelength and frequency) are known.

◆ A water wave travels at 7.5 m s^{-1} and has a frequency of 2.5 cycles per second (2.5 Hz or s^{-1}). What is its wavelength?

◆ Using Equation 2.4:

$$\text{wavelength (m)} = \frac{\text{speed (m s}^{-1}\text{)}}{\text{frequency (Hz or s}^{-1}\text{)}} = \frac{7.5 \text{ m s}^{-1}}{2.5 \text{ s}^{-1}} = 3.0 \text{ m}$$

The units of Hz and s^{-1} are interchangeable. Using s^{-1} on the top and bottom of this equation means they can be cancelled, leaving an answer in metres.

The wavelength of the water wave is 3.0 m. So there is a 3 metre distance between peaks of each wave.

It is a convention among scientists to describe colours by their wavelength measured in air. The wavelength of light in air is very short compared with wavelength values determined for water waves. The unit conventionally used to describe the wavelength of light is the nanometre (nm). Activity 2.1 (overleaf) allows you to calculate the wavelength of orange light using the same equation used above for a water wave. This calculation involves using large and small numbers expressed as powers of ten.

nm is short for nanometre and one nanometre is 10^{-9} m (or $\frac{1}{10^9}$) m.

Activity 2.1 Calculating the wavelength of light

Allow about 10 minutes

You may need a calculator.

This activity involves studying the example calculation below to determine the wavelength of turquoise (blue-green) light in air from Equation 2.4 (which you met in Box 2.2). Here we have added the units in which these quantities are measured to enable you to calculate an answer in nanometres (nm). Using the same steps, you can then calculate the wavelength of orange light in air.

Example calculation: calculating the wavelength of turquoise light

For turquoise light, the wave frequency is approximately 6×10^{14} Hz or s^{-1}.

The speed of light in air is very similar to the value in a vacuum (3×10^8 m s^{-1}) and this value can be used in the calculation.

Equation 2.4 is used to calculate the wavelength from the speed and frequency values.

$$\text{wavelength (m)} = \frac{\text{speed (m s}^{-1})}{\text{frequency (Hz or s}^{-1})} \qquad (2.4)$$

$$\text{wavelength (m)} = \frac{3 \times 10^8 \text{ m s}^{-1}}{6 \times 10^{14} \text{ s}^{-1}}$$

This equation can be simplified by considering separately the number and the 'power of ten' components of each term:

$$\text{wavelength (m)} = \frac{3}{6} \times \frac{10^8}{10^{14}}$$

which is the same as

$$\text{wavelength (m)} = 0.5 \times \frac{10^8}{10^{14}}$$

But how do you divide 10^8 by 10^{14}? Fortunately it's very simple.

For dividing powers of ten, the calculation involves *subtracting* the power of ten on the bottom of the fraction from the power of ten on the top, e.g.

$$\frac{10^8}{10^{14}} = 10^{(8-14)} = 10^{-6}$$

Therefore the wavelength (m) of turquoise light $= 0.5 \times 10^{(8-14)}$

$$\text{wavelength (m)} = 0.5 \times 10^{-6}$$

To convert from metres (m) into nanometres (10^{-9} m), you must multiply by 10^9. For multiplying powers of ten, the calculation involves simply adding together the individual powers of ten.

For example, $1000 \times 100 = 10^3 \times 10^2 = 10^{(3+2)} = 10^5 = 100\,000$

Therefore,

$$\text{wavelength} = (0.5 \times 10^{-6}) \times 10^9 \text{ nm}$$

$$\text{wavelength} = 0.5 \times 10^{(-6+9)} \text{ nm}$$

wavelength $= 0.5 \times 10^3$ nm $= 0.5 \times 1000$ nm

wavelength $= 500$ nm

The wavelength of turquoise light is 500 nm.

◆ Repeat the workings above to calculate the wavelength of orange light. (For orange light, the wave frequency is approximately 5×10^{14} Hz. The speed of light in air is 3×10^8 m s^{-1}.)

◆ The answer and the workings are shown in the comments on this activity at the end of the book.

While it is not necessary to memorise the wavelengths of specific colours, it is useful to know the wavelength at each extreme of the visible light range (violet and red colours):

Visible light of 400 nm wavelength corresponds to the colour violet. This is the shortest wavelength (and highest frequency) of visible light (Figure 2.5).

Visible light of 700 nm wavelength corresponds to the colour red. This is the longest wavelength (and lowest frequency) of visible light (Figure 2.5).

While it is helpful to consider light as an electromagnetic wave during transmission, the properties of light during other processes such as its absorption by atoms or molecules are better explained by describing light as a stream of particles. This way of explaining light as either a wave or a particle is called **wave–particle duality** (dew-al-it-ee) and arises because neither description is totally adequate to model all its known properties. However, both descriptions are connected in that a 'particle' or **photon** of light is regarded as a 'packet of energy' with the frequency of an electromagnetic wave. The energy of a photon can be calculated by multiplying a constant (a number known as Planck's constant) by the wave frequency. This is considered further in Chapter 5.

X-ray photons are explored in another book in this series, *Screening for Breast Cancer* (Parvin, 2007).

The remainder of this chapter studies the properties of light that lead to image formation within a camera, and then develops this further to study the process within the eye. In both examples, light will be considered as a stream of photons.

2.4 The eye as a camera

The eye is often compared to a camera because there are similarities in the way that the image is formed inside both of them.

Figure 2.10a (overleaf) shows a pinhole camera (which can be made from a box with a small hole in the front) located close to a candle. Light from a point at the top of the candle flame (labelled A in Figure 2.10b) is emitted in all possible directions. Notice that the walls of the box absorb light from point A preventing light from entering the box, apart from at the pinhole. Ideally the pinhole is so small that only a single tiny shaft of light from A gets into the box (such a tiny shaft of light is called a **light ray**, which traces the path that photons take from the candle, through the pinhole and into the camera).

The symbol ′ is known as a prime. A′ is pronounced as 'ay-prime'.

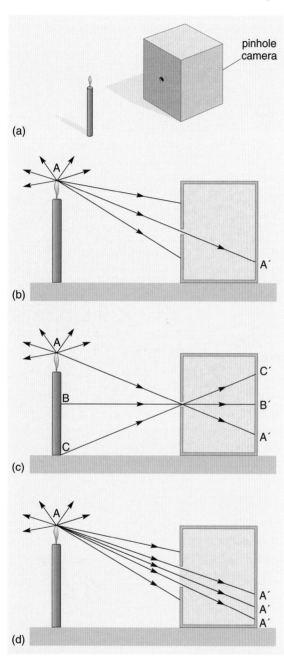

Figure 2.10 Principles of the pinhole camera. (a) Pinhole camera set-up. (b) Pinhole camera with small pinhole. The small size of the pinhole ensures that light from each point on the surface of the candle projects to only one point in the image on the back of the box. (c) Formation of an inverted image in a pinhole camera. (d) Pinhole camera with a large hole.

Light from point A entering through the pinhole can only reach the back of the box at one position (labelled A′ in Figure 2.10b). This is because light travels in a straight line. The same applies to each and every other point on the candle, as shown in Figure 2.10c. A single point in the outside world projects light to one, and only one, point at the back of this camera.

This light information is represented at the back of the box in the form of an **image**. An image is simply a two-dimensional map of the three-dimensional world and it has just two essential properties. First, each point in the three-dimensional world is represented by one, and only one, point in the image. Second, points in the image preserve the same spatial relationships as those between points in the world (i.e. they form the same shapes). In this pinhole camera, a picture is taken by placing light-sensitive photographic film at the back of the box. The eye is very similar in that the light-sensitive cells of the retina are at the back of the eye.

Note, however, that the image formed is *upside down*. For example, point A at the top of the candle flame is represented by A′ at the lowest point of the image. The image on the retina, as in the pinhole camera, forms upside down, but the brain learns to interpret it as the right way up. In individuals who are born blind but have sight restored in later life through surgery, the ability to see is not immediate after surgery. Such individuals find themselves initially unable to make much sense of their new sensory experience. The signals that reach the brain from the eye do not convey any meaningful information in themselves. It is only by *association* that they come to acquire meaning, and the brain has to learn how to interpret them. Interestingly it is possible to make goggles that invert the view so that the image forms on the retina the right way up, but the brain is so used to inverting the image that the wearer sees everything upside down. This is a bit disconcerting initially, but amazingly after about three days the brain makes the necessary adjustments and the wearer sees the world the right way up once again.

◆ Can you see one serious disadvantage of a pinhole camera?

◆ Pinhole cameras work by *excluding* most of the light from each point and so the image is inevitably dim.

Making the hole larger would cause problems, as shown in Figure 2.10d, because a cone-shaped shaft of light rays from each point could get into the box and light from each point in the world would project to a considerable area in the image. The image would thus be blurred.

Some early cameras worked on the pinhole principle and had to make up for this dimness of the image by collecting light over a considerable period of time. People in the photograph had to keep perfectly still during this time or they would appear in the photograph, if at all, as a streaky blur. This is clearly not a workable scenario for the human eye! The problem can be solved if use can be made of more of the rays of light coming from each point.

In the eye this is done by making the hole considerably larger, but manipulating the path of these extra light rays, so that rays from each point in the outside world are directed to just one point on the image at the back of the eye. This is possible because, under certain circumstances, light can be made to change its direction of travel using a transparent object known as a lens, which will be described later on. This deviation of the light path occurs when light passes from one medium to another, e.g. from air to glass, and is called **refraction** (Box 2.3).

Box 2.3 (Explanation) Refraction of light

Refraction is the process by which a light ray changes direction upon crossing an interface from one medium to another. To an observer, light appears to 'bend'. However, as light travels from an object to the eye in a straight line, bending cannot occur.

A good analogy to explain what happens is to imagine two lines of soldiers which represent a light ray (shown in green in Figure 2.11) marching on grass towards their sergeant major (with a red helmet). If the soldiers unexpectedly encounter a change of surface from grass to mud, their marching pace will change; soldiers travel slower across mud than grass. Therefore the line of soldiers that encounters the mud first will slow down before the other line. This causes the marching arrangement to pivot at the grass–mud interface and change direction, because the soldiers are trained to march side by side. Refraction has the same effect and results from a change in the speed of light as photons pass from one medium to another. Photons at one side of a light ray will change speed before photons at the other side, changing the direction of the light ray as with the two lines of soldiers.

Refraction occurs in a prism or the lens of a camera because the speed of light is less in glass than in air. The curved surface of the lens provides an angled interface to control this change in direction precisely for all light rays entering the camera.

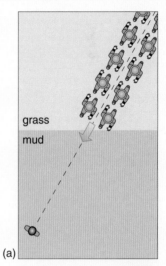

(a)

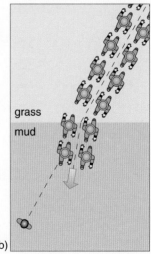

(b)

Figure 2.11 A demonstration of refraction with marching soldiers. (a) The soldiers are marching across grass towards their sergeant major, with a red helmet. (b) They encounter mud which slows one marching line before the other. Part (c) of this diagram appears overleaf.

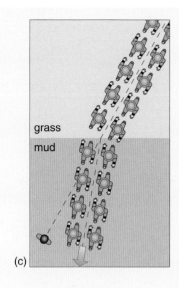

(c)

(c) Having crossed from grass to mud, the soldiers now travel in a new direction.

Figure 2.12 shows a more sophisticated camera fitted with a lens. Rays of light from the candle travel through the air until they reach the lens. As there is now a large opening at the front of the camera many light rays can reach the back of the camera, making the image brighter. The lens redirects all the light rays from the top of the candle flame (point D) to its respective image position at the back of the camera (D′) without blurring. To achieve this effect, the refraction process must be controlled by a transparent object of exactly the right shape. This shape is that of a *convex* lens, as shown in Box 2.4.

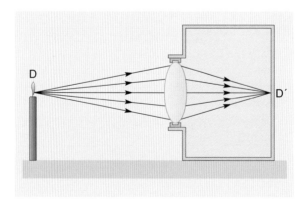

Figure 2.12 A camera with a (convex) lens, showing that light rays from point D are changed in direction to project to a single point at the back of the camera, D′.

Box 2.4 (Explanation) Convex lenses

The most familiar lens shape is **convex**. Two convex lenses are shown in Figure 2.13. In each lens, the centre is thicker than the top and bottom extremities. The smooth curvature of a lens is very important to ensure that light rays are precisely refracted at each part of the lens. This smoothness redirects rays, in this case with matching orientations (known as parallel rays) so that they pass through the lens and meet at a single point beyond (known as the **principal focal point**). The thickness of the lens changes the position of this principal focal point, with a thin convex lens forming a principal focal point at a greater distance than a thick convex lens (Figure 2.13).

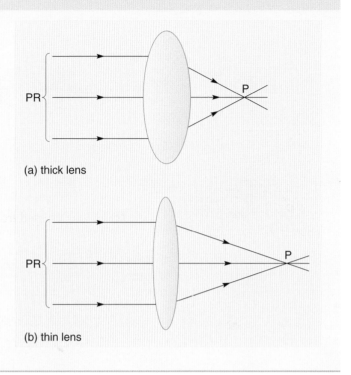

(a) thick lens

(b) thin lens

Figure 2.13 Two convex lenses: (a) thick and (b) thin. The thick lens changes the direction of the light rays more than the thin lens. P = principal focal point; PR = parallel rays.

Using a lens will make the image much brighter, but solving one problem has caused another! Unfortunately, the camera lens system depicted in Figure 2.12 only works for objects at one particular distance. If the object is closer than this, as shown in Figure 2.14, or further away, the light from each point no longer projects to a single point at the back of the camera. The image is no longer *sharp*; it is blurred. This presents a dilemma: a small hole (in a pinhole camera) allows an image to remain in focus over a wide range of distances but produces a dim image; a large hole (in a camera with a lens) produces a brighter image but this is only sharp for objects at a limited range of distances. Good vision requires the eye to generate images that are both bright and sharp for a wide range of distances.

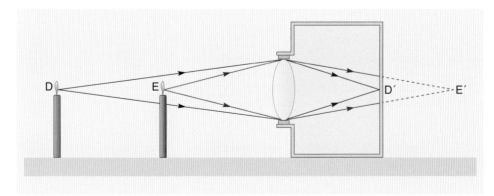

Figure 2.14 A camera with a lens photographing two objects at different distances. Light rays from point D project to a single point on the back of the camera, D′. Light rays originating from other distances (such as point E) do not project to a single point, and as a result appear blurred. E′ shows where a sharp image would be formed if the back of the camera was not in the way.

This dilemma is resolved in the eye by introducing two refinements. First, there is a variable sized hole, the pupil, through which light enters: in dim light the pupil opens up to admit as much light as possible, whereas in bright light it closes down to a pinhole. This has the effect of making objects remain in focus over a greater range of distances. This opening and closing of the pupil is an automatic, or *reflex*, response (Box 2.5). Doctors and paramedics use a small torch to shine a bright light into the eye of someone who is unconscious to check whether their reflex reactions are operating normally.

The nervous system is explored in another book in this series, *Pain* (Toates, 2007).

Box 2.5 (Explanation) Pupil size

Smooth muscle is found in the iris of the eye (Figure 2.2). The nerve signals controlling smooth muscle do not come from the regions of the brain that process information and plan actions, but come from the autonomic nervous system (ANS), a largely 'automatic' or 'self-governing' system. The smooth muscle of the iris is arranged into two layers: a circular layer which when contracted reduces the size of the pupil, and a layer of muscle fibres that radiate out from the inner rim of the annulus so that their contraction increases, or dilates, pupil size. The size of the pupil varies predominantly in response to environmental lighting levels. But the muscles of the iris also respond to more general 'commands' from the ANS. For example, on emotional occasions the ANS causes the pupil to dilate. So you may be able to tell whether someone is romantically interested in you by the size of their pupils!

The second refinement is in the lens of the eye. This is a refinement, rather than a strict necessity, because most of the light refraction takes place at the cornea, the transparent tissue covering the front of the eye. The function of the lens is to allow some flexibility in focusing (by changing the position of the principal focal point). The lens is an elastic structure that can vary its thickness and curvature. This is achieved by the lens being suspended by ligaments that are attached to muscles, known as ciliary muscles which control the tension (Figure 2.15).

To bring distant objects into focus, the lens must be pulled flat. This is achieved when the ciliary muscles relax and the suspensory ligaments are taut, pulling the lens flat (Figure 2.15a). To bring closer objects into focus, the lens must be more curved (Figure 2.15b), so the ciliary muscles contract, releasing the tension on the ligaments that hold the lens in place and allowing the lens to bulge into its natural shape.

This process of changing the lens shape to focus on objects at different distances is called **accommodation**.

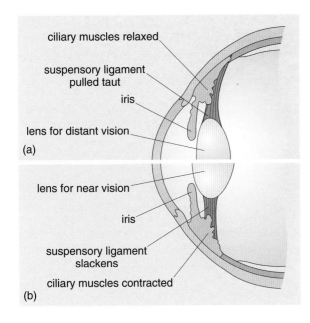

(a)

(b)

Figure 2.15
Accommodation. (a) Tension in the suspensory ligaments pulls the lens flat so that its curvature decreases, light is refracted less and distant objects are in focus. (b) Tension is released in the ligaments so that the lens bulges to its natural shape. Curvature increases and light is refracted more, so nearby objects are in focus.

Activity 2.2 Lenses and focusing

Allow about 1 hour

Activity 2.2 is a multimedia exercise on the DVD associated with this book that looks in detail at the properties of convex lenses. The eye contains two convex structures – the cornea and the lens. Interactive exercises demonstrate how convex structures process light, providing an insight into the workings of the front of the eye. There are some short interactive questions based on the exercises which you can answer 'on screen'.

The activity introduces the **focal length**. This is the distance (in metres) from the centre of the lens to the principal focal point.

If you are unable to complete this activity now, do it as soon as possible.

Please note that the 'Introduction' menu option shows a very short video clip of an eye dissection on abattoir tissue from a horse; watching this exercise is optional for those uncomfortable with viewing surgical procedures.

2.5 Light-sensitive cells in the retina

Early cameras captured images on photographic plates containing chemicals sensitive to light (*photosensitive* chemicals). The retina performs a similar function in the eye because it contains receptor cells which are photosensitive. The retina is composed of many cell layers as shown in Figure 2.16a and b overleaf. Light, travelling through the vitreous humour, strikes the retina and travels through several layers of retinal cells *before* it strikes the visual receptor cells called **rods** and **cones** (Figure 2.16c shows a rod in more detail). There are around 125 million visual receptor cells in the retina (also known as *photoreceptors*). Having two types of photoreceptor rather than one allows the eye to work over a wider range of lighting levels than one type would allow. However, both rods and cones only

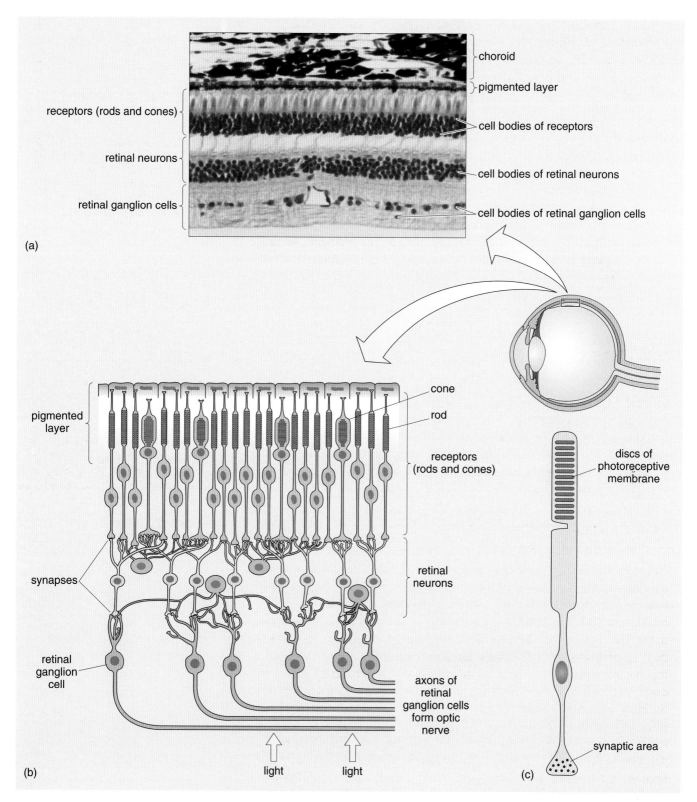

Figure 2.16 (a) Photomicrograph of a cross-section of the human retina magnified about a thousand times (Source: Biophoto Associates/Science Photo Library). (b) Diagrammatic cross-section of the retina showing how light must pass through several cell layers comprising first the retinal ganglion cells, then several layers of retinal neurons, before reaching the rods and cones. The region where one cell communicates with another is known as a synapse. (c) Diagram of a rod photoreceptor.

detect light in the visible region of the electromagnetic spectrum (between about 400 and 700 nm). Rods are very sensitive and function best under poor light conditions, for instance at night, whereas cones work best under bright daylight conditions and are also responsible for colour vision (the subject of Chapter 3). Rods outnumber cones by about 20:1 and are about 1000 times more sensitive to light.

The rods and cones are embedded in a pigmented layer (Figure 2.16a and b). This pigmented layer, known as retinal pigmented epithelium (RPE), lies next to the choroid. Both the choroid and the RPE contain the black-coloured pigment melanin which absorbs light that has not been captured by the rods and cones. Melanin thus prevents the remaining light from being reflected off the back of the eye and interfering with the production of a clear image on the retina. Visual pigments contained within rods and cones absorb, and thereby detect, the incoming light. When visible light is absorbed by the pigments, there is a chemical change in these molecules (to be described in Chapter 3) which triggers a cascade of events, eventually generating an electrical change within the receptor cell. This change can be communicated to other cells nearby and there is an initial processing of visual information in the retina (see Box 2.6). Finally, retinal ganglion cells carry the processed information to the brain, with long thin projections of these cells (called axons) forming the optic nerve (Figure 2.16b).

A pigment is a molecule that gives a tissue a characteristic colour. 'Retinal' is the adjective applied to structures in the retina. It is also the name of the visual pigment (as described in Chapter 3).

A nerve is a bundle of axons.

Box 2.6 (Explanation) Processing in the retina

Cells are constantly sending and receiving signals across their outer membranes. Cells of the nervous system, called *neurons*, are particularly active in this way; in fact, it is their chief role. Neurons are located in the brain and in other regions of the nervous system, including the retina of the eye. Rods and cones (the photoreceptors) communicate with retinal neurons by releasing molecules known as *neurotransmitters*. The junctions between these communicating cells of the nervous system are known as *synapses*. (Figure 2.16b)

Neurotransmitters move across the synaptic gap (the gap between communicating neurons) and influence the recipient (i.e. post-synaptic) cell, causing it to alter its electrical activity. There are many synapses on each retinal neuron, so each cell is receiving lots of little pieces of information in the form of chemical signals. Whatever the outcome, this cell will itself be in communication with others, through thousands of synapses. From this you may deduce that each photoreceptor cell will have the ability to exert some influence on a considerable population of neurons in the retina. So there is an initial processing of information within the retina. Thus the information that leaves the retina, carried by retinal ganglion cells (the only retinal neurons to have long axons), is transmitted in precisely ordered patterns along nerves that act like dedicated routes from the eye to various regions of the brain. Information about colour, shape and movement is carried in different information streams and is further analysed within specific and different areas of the brain.

Neurons are cells in the brain and nervous system that have a communication function and are discussed more fully in another book in this series (Toates, 2007)

The radius is the distance from any point on the rim of a circle to the centre of the circle.

μm is the symbol for a micrometre (one millionth of a metre)

Rods and cones are differently distributed throughout the retina. When the retina is examined using special equipment (Figure 2.17a), a yellow area with a radius of about 2 mm, called the **macula lutea** (mak-ue-lah loo-tee-ah) (or yellow spot) can be seen (Figure 2.17b). At the centre of the macula lutea is a small depression called the **fovea** (foh-vee-ah) (look back at Figure 2.3), an area with a radius of 250 μm consisting exclusively of cones packed tightly together. The other retinal cells are pulled aside from the fovea so that light has nothing to impede its path to the cones and can form the sharpest possible image. From the fovea, a signal from each cone is kept *separate* so that it is possible to discriminate fine detail, and thus provide clear, distinct vision. By contrast, the output from rods is pooled.

◆ What is the disadvantage of pooling the information from many rods?

◆ If the information from many rods is combined they cannot be used to discriminate fine detail.

There are no photoreceptor cells where the optic nerve leaves the back of the eye. So this area is called the *blind spot* (see Figure 2.3). Activity 2.3 is a demonstration of your blind spot.

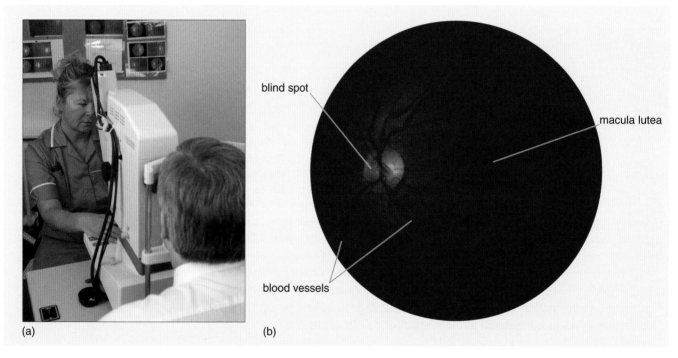

(a) (b)

Figure 2.17   (a) A retinal screening technician photographing the back of the eye with a digital camera. (Source: Open University). (b) Photograph of a retina viewed through the pupil. Using this technology, the macula lutea normally appears dark. (Source: Joy Wilson/Boots Opticians).

Activity 2.3   The blind spot

Allow about 5 minutes

You can demonstrate your own blind spot by carrying out the following test. Below is an image of a filled circular dot and a bold plus sign. Now close your right eye, and focus your left eye on the bold plus sign while holding the page at arm's length. You should be able to see both symbols. Slowly bring the page closer to your eyes while still focusing on the cross.

At some point the dot vanishes. This demonstrates your blind spot. It occurs where the light rays from the dot are focused when the dot vanishes. (If you continue moving the page closer to your face, the dot reappears.)

Visual information carried from the eyes by the optic nerve reaches a region of the brain called the *primary visual cortex*. (This is found in the occipital lobe of the brain, which is at the very back of the head; see Figure 2.18). When relaxing in a comfortable chair, the surface of skull pressed into the headrest corresponds well to the region of skull overlaying the occipital lobe. The primary visual cortex processes nerve signals around 25 times a second (i.e. a frequency of 25 Hz). As with watching a film at the cinema, these updated 'snapshots' can be synthesised by the brain to create the perception of smooth movement.

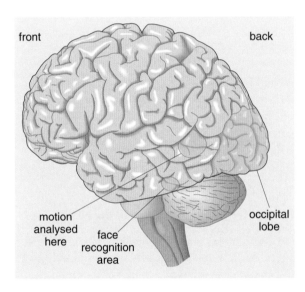

Figure 2.18   The brain showing the occipital lobe where the primary visual cortex is located, and two specialised areas, the area where motion is analysed and the area where faces are recognised.

In addition to recognising shapes and movement within the visual field, retinal processing of information about colour is the first stage of colour perception. The next chapter looks in more detail at the science of colour vision.

Summary of Chapter 2

2.1   The eye is protected by a number of structures: the bony skull, cushioning fatty tissues, eyebrows, eyelids and lashes. Tears are also protective.

2.2   Light is an electromagnetic wave which travels in a straight line and can be described in terms of its wavelength or frequency.

2.3   Visible light is the region of the electromagnetic spectrum that the eye can detect. The visible region extends from wavelengths of approximately 400 nm (violet) to 700 nm (red).

2.4 Light can also be thought of as a stream of packets of energy, known as photons.

2.5 The eye operates like a camera in the way it forms an image on the retina at the back of the eye.

2.6 The pupil can vary in size to allow more or less light into the eye.

2.7 Refraction is the process where light changes direction upon crossing an interface between two different media. This process occurs at the cornea and lens of the eye.

2.8 The cornea and lens have a convex shape and thus refract light rays to produce a sharply focused image on the retina.

2.9 Most of the focusing occurs at the cornea; the lens can alter shape to 'fine tune' the focusing of the image – a process known as accommodation.

2.10 The retina contains two types of photoreceptor cells: rods and cones. Rods are more sensitive to light, they outnumber cones 20:1 and are distributed over most of the retina except the central region, but cannot perceive colour. Cones detect colour and allow vision of fine detail. They are concentrated at the fovea.

2.11 Information from the rods and cones is processed by neurons in the retina, and is then passed along the optic nerve to the brain where different areas analyse different aspects of visual perception.

Learning outcomes for Chapter 2

After studying this chapter and its associated activities, you should be able to:

LO 2.1 Define and use in context, or recognise definitions and applications of, each of the terms printed in **bold** in the text. (Questions 2.1 and 2.4)

LO 2.2 Identify the basic anatomy and protective structures of the human eye. (Question 2.2)

LO 2.3 Describe the electromagnetic spectrum and use the equation relating the speed, wavelength and frequency of a wave to perform simple calculations. (Question 2.3 and Activity 2.1)

LO 2.4 Relate the design of a camera to the anatomy of the eye and describe how an image is formed inside a camera or the eye. (Question 2.4 and DVD Activity 2.2)

LO 2.5 Describe how the process of accommodation assists clear vision of objects close up or far away. (Question 2.5 and DVD Activity 2.2)

LO 2.6 Describe the structure of the retina, and the properties and distribution of the retinal photoreceptor cells. (Question 2.6 and Activity 2.3)

LO 2.7 Identify some of the structures involved in processing visual information in the retina and the brain. (Question 2.7)

Self-assessment questions for Chapter 2

You also had the opportunity to demonstrate LOs 2.4 and 2.5 by completing DVD Activity 2.2.

Question 2.1 (LOs 2.1 and 2.4)

There is a medical condition called a detached retina, where the retina no longer stays in place at the back of the eyeball and moves around. What effect will this have on vision?

Question 2.2 (LO 2.2)

While you are cycling on a bike, an insect flies towards your eye. How might your eye respond to protect itself?

Question 2.3 (LO 2.3)

A suntan (and also sunburn!) is caused by ultraviolet radiation. How does the frequency (and wavelength) of ultraviolet radiation relate to that of visible light?

Question 2.4 (LOs 2.1 and 2.4)

Name the components of the eye that correspond to the following parts of the pinhole camera and explain their purpose: (a) pinhole; (b) front wall of the camera box; (c) back wall of the camera box.

Question 2.5 (LO 2.5)

You wave goodbye to relatives on board a train as it leaves the station platform. What is happening to the thickness of the lens in your eye as you watch the train travel into the distance? What structures are involved in producing this effect?

Question 2.6 (LO 2.6)

What black-coloured pigment absorbs any extraneous light within the eye that is not captured by the photoreceptor cells? Why is this important?

Question 2.7 (LO 2.7)

In an accident, a person suffers traumatic injury to the back of the brain. Is it possible that vision could be impaired following this brain injury?

CHAPTER 3

COLOUR VISION AND COLOUR DEFICIENCIES

3.1 Introduction

Worldwide, around 8% of men (but almost no women) experience some level of **colour deficiency**; they find it difficult to distinguish certain colours, most commonly red and green. This can deny people access to certain jobs (see Table 3.1), and in some countries to a driving licence. In a few instances, people are **colour blind** – they can see no colour at all. In this chapter, we explore the interaction of visible light with the receptors in the eye to create colour vision and describe what has gone wrong in colour deficiency.

Table 3.1 Jobs not open to people with colour deficiencies. (Source: http://www.kent.ac.uk/careers/disabled.htm)

- commercial airline pilots, air traffic controllers, airport technical and maintenance staff
- engineers and signal engineers, and aircraft pilots in the armed services
- train drivers, railway engineers, maintenance staff and trackside workers
- naval officers, merchant navy officers and all ranks engaged in watch keeping duties, and all submarine personnel
- Customs and Excise officers
- some engineers, e.g. electrical
- workers in industrial colour quality control and colour matching
- fine art reproduction work
  (and in some cases police, photography, printing, and design and fashion jobs*)

* Added by author.

3.2 Absorption and reflection of wavelengths

As you saw in Section 2.2, electromagnetic radiation consists of a spectrum of all wavelengths, with visible light from 400 to 700 nm being detected by the eye. If the visible light passes though a glass prism, it is separated out into all the different wavelengths and we perceive them as a 'rainbow' of colours. This was first observed by Sir Isaac Newton in 1672 who initially named only five colours: red, yellow, green, blue, and violet. He later included orange and indigo to make it seven, to tie in with the number of notes in a musical scale. These colours are the ones you see as a natural phenomenon in a rainbow, when the raindrops act as prisms refracting the light (Figure 3.1). Most western cultures still traditionally cite the seven colours of the rainbow, probably because seven is thought to be a lucky number; in practice, it is difficult to distinguish the different colours at the blue end of the spectrum, particularly indigo.

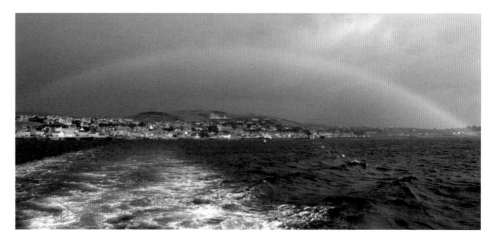

Figure 3.1   A rainbow over Stromness harbour. (Source: John McGill)

Human eyes are able to distinguish different wavelengths and interpret them in terms of colour, but they do so by working in the opposite way to a prism. A prism splits up the light into its constituent wavelengths which we see as a rainbow of colours, whereas the visual system (eye and brain) *merges* the effect of all wavelengths received and interprets them as a composite colour. The colours that you perceive are due to the way in which the receptors in the retina process the information. Because there is reduced ability to distinguish between different wavelengths at the blue end of the spectrum, it is quite common for instance for one person to describe an object as 'green' when someone else sees it as 'blue'. The language of colour demonstrates the fact that colour is perceived and is not the same for everyone. The maximum number of basic colour terms in any language seems to be 12 (in Russian, which distinguishes two types of blue). English uses 11 terms: white, black, grey, red, orange, yellow, green, blue, purple, pink and brown. Many languages use fewer terms: Navaho, for instance, does not distinguish blue and green; Japanese uses 'awo' for green, blue or 'pale' depending on context; and Hanunóo (Philippines) uses only black, white, red and green.

The colour of the everyday objects you see around you results from the two processes of *absorption* and *reflection* (already described in Chapter 2). When visible light hits an object, some of the wavelengths in the light are absorbed by the molecules in the object because they interact with the electrons in these molecules. The wavelengths that are not absorbed are reflected and thence fall on the eye and are detected. If *all* the light hitting an object is absorbed then that object appears black to a viewer. The combination of the reflected frequencies gives the perceived colour of the object. If no wavelengths are absorbed but all are reflected, the object appears white.

Scientific instruments, known as spectrometers (spect-rom-etters), are able to analyse the colours of transparent and solid objects by quantitatively measuring the proportion of visible light that is absorbed at each wavelength. This value is known as *absorbance*. These values can then be plotted as a graph showing the absorbance on a vertical axis against wavelength on the horizontal axis. Figure 3.2

shows such a graph; it is known as an *absorption spectrum*. The example in Figure 3.2 shows the absorption of light by a transparent solution of blue dye. Visible light is passed through the solution, and the amount of light of each wavelength absorbed is shown as a black silhouette against the spectrum of visible light. Notice that the light absorbed is predominantly at the red and orange end of the visible spectrum, and that the combination of blue, green and yellow wavelengths not absorbed is detected by the eye and *perceived* as blue.

Any plot of absorbance versus wavelength or frequency is known as a spectrum. It is usually distinguished by labelling the region of the electromagnetic spectrum covered. So here you would refer to a 'visible spectrum'.

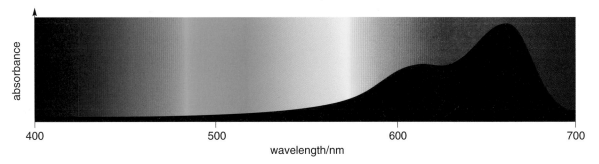

Figure 3.2   Absorption spectrum of a blue dye set against the visible spectrum of sunlight.

For opaque objects, something slightly different happens; some wavelengths are absorbed by the object, and the remainder are reflected by the surface and then detected by the eye. It is these reflected wavelengths that determine the colour of the object. Figure 3.3 demonstrates why a ripe tomato appears red. The spectrum shows that the tomato absorbs the wavelengths at the blue end of the spectrum, thus leaving the remaining wavelengths to be reflected and detected by the eye, which perceives them as the colour red.

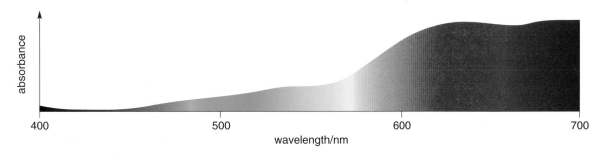

Figure 3.3   Reflection spectrum from the skin of a ripe tomato.

3.3   Mixing colours

3.3.1   Colours

As will become clear in Section 3.4, in order to understand how colour is detected at the retina of the eye, you first need to learn a little about the processes of mixing and adding the colours of light.

The three primary colours when mixing light are red, green and blue (Section 3.3.2). By extending the range of colours and arranging them to form a colour circle as shown in Figure 3.4, every colour on the circle can be described in terms of its two neighbouring unique hues, i.e. orange is a yellowish red, and purple is a bluish red. The colours on *opposite sides* of the circle are said to be **complementary colours**; thus yellow is complementary to violet and red is complementary to cyan. Cyan is the colour perceived when red is removed from white light.

◆ What colour of light is perceived when blue is removed from white light?

◆ Orange.

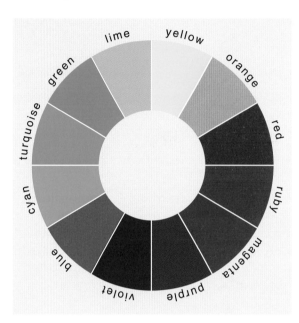

Figure 3.4 The colour circle; the colours on opposite sides of the circle are said to be *complementary*.

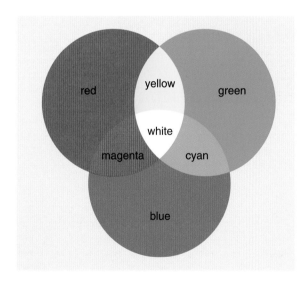

Figure 3.5 Additive primary colours red, green and blue combining in pairs to give yellow, magenta and cyan, and all three to give white.

3.3.2 The additive primary colours

If you mix together red, green and blue light, then where all three colours overlap white is seen. These three colours are known as the **additive primary colours**. Where these three primary colours overlap in pairs, a second set of three colours – yellow, magenta and cyan, the *subtractive primaries*, is found (Figure 3.5). By varying the intensity of the overlapping spots, *any* colour in the visible spectrum can be produced; this phenomenon is known as **trichromacy** (try-crow-mah-see) (from the Latin *tri* meaning three and the Greek *chroma* meaning colour) because of the three primary colours. As you will see in Section 3.4, it is this property that is used in the retina to detect the colour of an object from its reflected wavelengths.

You may have already said to yourself: 'but if I mix red and green paint, I don't get yellow, I get brown', and indeed you are correct. The above paragraph refers to the mixing of different wavelengths of *visible light*, which is important in the context of colour vision, but does not apply to the mixing of paints, dyes and pigments. For that you need to turn to the subtractive primaries, and if you are interested these are explained in Box 3.1.

Box 3.1 (Enrichment) Printing inks

If you buy cartridges of inks for an inkjet printer (Figure 3.6a), the three colours used are yellow, magenta and cyan, known as the *subtractive primaries* (Figure 3.6b). Why aren't red, green and blue used? Think of one ink, cyan for example, printed on white paper (Figure 3.6c). It absorbs the red wavelengths, corresponding to the *complementary colour*, from the sunlight leaving the green and blue wavelengths to be reflected and observed by the eye. If you now think of yellow ink printed alone, the blue wavelengths are absorbed and red and green reflected. If both cyan and

yellow are printed, then both the red *and* the blue wavelengths are absorbed, leaving only green to be reflected (Figure 3.6b and c). Thus by mixing the correct proportions of the subtractive primaries, all colours can be produced. If you try doing this by using additive primaries, it will not work; unlike the subtractive primaries which are composite colours, the additive primaries reflect pure colours of a much smaller wavelength range (once the complementary colour has been absorbed, there is little left to be reflected).

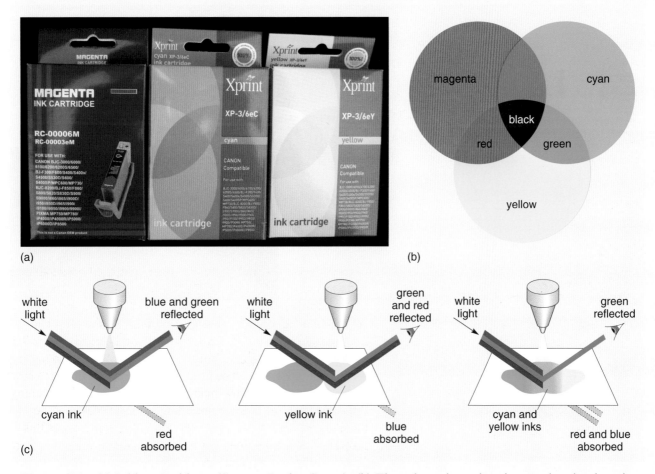

(a)

(b)

(c)

Figure 3.6 (a) Inkjet cartridges. (Source: Lesley Smart). (b) The subtractive primaries overlapping in pairs. (c) Printing yellow on cyan gives green.

3.4 Detection of light by the eye

3.4.1 The structure of the retina

You saw in Section 2.5 that the retina is the detection apparatus at the back of the eye. It is a tissue composed of many layers. To recap, there are around 125 million photoreceptors of two types, rods and cones, allowing the eye to work over a very wide range of light intensities from the dimmest starlight to bright sunlight. Rods outnumber cones by about 20:1 and are about 1000 times more sensitive to light. There is only one type of rod cell and they provide only black and white or *monochromatic* vision (under dim light conditions, e.g. at night, you see only in black and white). However, there are *three different types* of cone cells, which work best under bright daylight conditions. By using the principles of the trichromacy theory, we are able to understand how the three different cones allow colour vision (see Section 3.5).

Cones are densely packed in the central fovea region of the retina where there are no rods (Figure 3.7a). At the fovea, all of the other cell types are squeezed out of the way (the 'foveal pit'), allowing maximum light to hit the cones (Figure 3.7b).

The area in and around the fovea has a pale yellow pigmentation contained in the retinal ganglion cells – the macula lutea (see Section 2.5); damage to this area can cause significant eyesight problems (known as *macular degeneration*) in later life, as you will see in Section 6.3.

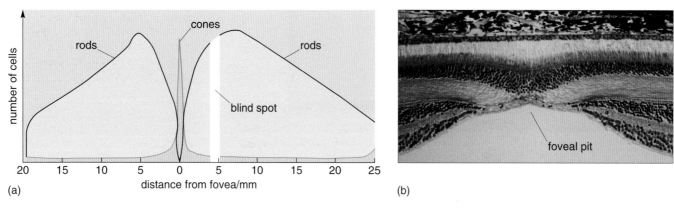

Figure 3.7 (a) Distribution of rods and cones in the retina. (b) Electron micrograph of the foveal pit showing cell layers pushed to one side. (Source: Gene Cox/Science Photo Library)

3.4.2 From retina to optic nerve

You saw in Section 3.2 how objects absorb some of the visible wavelengths falling on them, reflecting the remainder and thus imparting colour. It is the molecules on the surface of objects that carry out this process. (Box 3.2 contains a short introduction to molecules and chemical bonding.) Coloured pigments contained within rods and cones are known as *photopigments*. Photopigments absorb particular wavelengths of light; it is by virtue of their structure that they are particularly good at doing this. The photopigment in a rod cell consists of *cis*-retinal (structure **1** and Figure 3.8a) attached to a protein called opsin. (In this molecule the carbon atoms attached to each of the circled carbons are on the *same* side of the double bond (*cis*).) The pigments in the three different types of cone cells also consist of *cis*-retinal but each has attached a slightly different opsin molecule.

Cis- (pronounced, 'siss') is Latin for 'on the same side' and is the opposite of *trans*, which means 'on the opposite side'.

1 *cis*-retinal

When light is absorbed by the *cis*-retinal molecule, the energy imparted by the light moves (excites) the electrons in the double bonds, causing the molecule to change shape at one carbon atom (structure **2** and Figure 3.8b): the number and type of the atoms are exactly the same, but the shape changes – at the circled double bond, the end of the chain swings round from the bent position to form a linear chain; this is known as the *trans-* form of retinal. (In *trans*-retinal the carbon atoms attached to each of the circled carbons are on *opposite* sides of the double bond.)

2 *trans*-retinal

Notice that in these large molecules it is conventional to group similar atoms together, as in CH$_3$ here, rather than drawing all the individual bonds. It makes diagrams less crowded and gives more emphasis to the important bonds.

Once the light has brought about the chemical change from *cis-* to *trans*-retinal, this in turn triggers a change in the shape of the attached protein, opsin, and thence a further cascade of events, eventually generating an electrical signal which is processed by the retinal neuron cells, and thence to the retinal ganglion cells which send the signals to the brain via the optic nerve. The *trans*-retinal, which becomes a free molecule during these reactions, finally converts back into the *cis-* form and reattaches to the opsin, and the whole process can begin again.

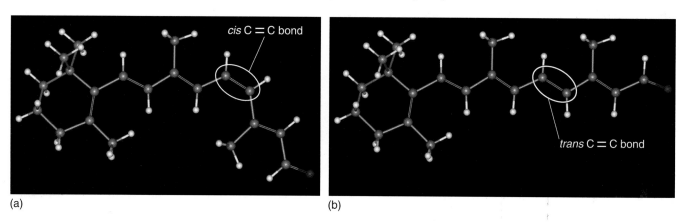

(a)   (b)

Figure 3.8 Computer models of: (a) *cis*-retinal and (b) *trans*-retinal. (Source: Accelrys)

Box 3.2 (Explanation) Atoms, molecules and bonding

Atoms are made up of several different sorts of smaller particles; important for our purposes are protons and electrons. The **atomic nucleus** contains **protons**, each of which carries a unit of *positive* electric charge; the atoms of different elements have differing numbers of protons. An atomic nucleus is surrounded by **electrons**, each one of which possesses a unit of *negative* charge, thus balancing the charges on the protons. Each element has been assigned a **chemical symbol**: for instance, H stands for hydrogen, C for carbon, F for fluorine and O for oxygen.

Different elements react with each other to form **compounds**. For example, water, H_2O, is formed from hydrogen and oxygen: the atoms form chemical **bonds** with each other. Atoms form bonds with other atoms by using their outermost electrons (the inner electrons are tightly bound to the nucleus and so are unavailable for bonding). One of the important types of bonding is known as *covalent*, where one of the outer or bonding electrons from each of two adjacent atoms is shared between the two atoms, forming a single electron-pair bond, or **covalent bond**. This type of bonding is used in forming **molecules**. The hydrogen atom, for example, possesses only one electron. Two hydrogen atoms each share an electron to make a molecule with a single covalent bond:

$$H \; {}^{\text{x}}_{\text{x}} \; H$$

where x represents the hydrogen electron.

This is often depicted as H—H, where the straight line denotes the covalent bond. The number of electrons available for bonding varies from element to element. An oxygen atom is able to share *two* electrons with other atoms, for instance forming the carbon dioxide, CO_2, molecule, with *double* bonds depicted as O=C=O. Carbon has *four* outer electrons involved in bonding, and carbon-to-carbon double bonds, C=C, are also found in many molecules in which the two C atoms are connected to other atoms such as O and H, as in structures **1** and **2**.

Molecules containing only carbon-to-carbon single bonds, C—C, can change their shape easily. However, the presence of a carbon-to-carbon double bond, C=C, in a molecule makes that part of the molecule rigid. Consider the shape of butene, a small flat molecule; it can adopt two possible shapes:

3   **4**

Both structures **3** and **4** have the same numbers of atoms, but different inflexible shapes; they are said to be *isomers*.

◆ Which isomer is *cis*-butene and which is *trans*-butene?

◆ Structure **3** is the *cis*-isomer where the carbon atoms attached to the double bond are on the same side of the double bond. In structure **4** the carbon atoms attached to the double bond are opposite each other, so this molecule is the *trans*-isomer.

Vitamin A

The *cis*-retinal in the retina is made from vitamin A. An early symptom of vitamin A deficiency is night blindness. Vitamin A deficiency in pregnant women can cause night blindness and may also increase the risk of maternal mortality during or soon after childbirth. This can be effectively and inexpensively cured by taking a vitamin A supplement.

In developing countries, particularly those with rice-based diets and a lack of vegetables, poor nutrition commonly causes vitamin A deficiency. It is distressing to discover that a deficiency of vitamin A, together with measles, is the main cause of child blindness worldwide. Both can be prevented. These children often die young because vitamin A deficiency also makes them susceptible to infections.

Childhood blindness is preventable in the majority of cases, and its incidence has been reduced through programmes that combine the elimination of vitamin A deficiency with immunisation against measles through the Global Child Survival Partnership (WHO, 2007b).

3.5 Seeing in colour

3.5.1 The three cones: S, M and L

If humans had different receptors in their eyes for every possible colour, the number of receptors responsive to any particular colour, say orange, would have to be low because of space constraints, and the eye's sensitivity to orange light would be very much less than to visible light. In practice, however, the eye's sensitivity to separate colours is almost as good as it is to visible light. This is because there are only three types of colour receptor in the eye, one sensitive to red wavelengths, one to green and one to blue. Humans are said to be *trichromats*, and their ability to see in colour is explained by the trichromacy theory of the three additive primaries (Section 3.2). The colour perceived depends on the relative extent to which each of the three colour receptors is stimulated. Finally, colour is 'synthesised' or 'perceived' in specific areas within the brain.

The three colour receptors are the three different types of cone cell, each containing a slightly modified pigment (Section 3.4.2) which causes them to absorb light of slightly different wavelengths (Figure 3.9). The S-cones are sensitive to light of the shortest wavelengths, in the blue–violet region of the spectrum, with maximum sensitivity at 420 nm. M-cones respond in the green region (maximum sensitivity at 534 nm); and the L-cones respond to the yellow and red wavelengths (maximum sensitivity at 564 nm).

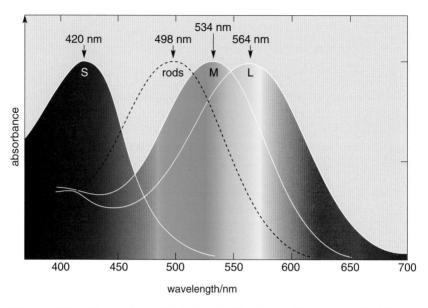

Figure 3.9 Absorption of light by the S-, M- and L- cone cells (the response curve for rod cells is shown as a dotted line).

◆ S, M and L stand for short, medium and long (wavelength). The cones are also commonly known as blue, green, and red respectively.

◆ If light of red and green wavelengths reaches the eye, what colour will be perceived? (Hint: look at Figure 3.5.)

◆ The L- and M-cones in the retina will be stimulated, respectively, and the brain will interpret this as yellow.

Notice that the response ranges (shown by the curves) of the three cones overlap, a necessity for the trichromacy theory to be able to work and create all possible colours.

There is only *one* type of rod cell, with maximum response at 498 nm, i.e. in the middle of the visible wavelength region (Figure 3.9). Because there is only one type, rods cannot discriminate different colours and are sensitive only to the intensity of light.

3.5.2   Colour deficiencies

As stated at the beginning of this chapter, approximately 8% of men, but very few women, have colour deficiencies, most commonly red/green colour deficiency. The problem usually lies in a faulty gene which is inherited from the mother, but the condition can also be caused by disease or injury.

The trichromacy theory provides the explanation for the different types of colour deficiency. In the majority of cases, the problem lies in the fact that one of the types of cone responds to slightly different wavelengths from normal. In about

5% of males, the M-cone response curve moves to longer wavelengths nearer to the L-cone response curve (Figure 3.10), bringing the 'red' and 'green' detectors into close proximity so that a fine discrimination between the two colours cannot be made. In 1% of males, the L-cone response curve moves to shorter wavelengths, with the same effect.

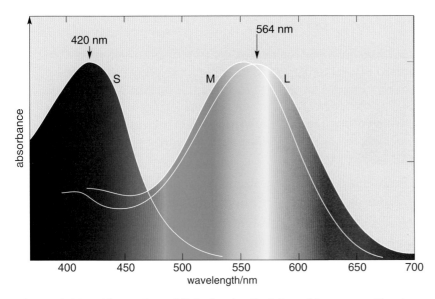

Figure 3.10 Absorption of light by the S-, M- and L- cone cells where the M-cone curve has moved to longer wavelengths.

In some men, one or more types of cone cell does not work or is missing; about 1–2% of males lack either the M- or the L-cones. If the L-cones are faulty or absent, the eyes will still respond to blue, green, yellow and orange, and even orange–red light as covered by the first two response curves in Figure 3.9; however, it will be impossible to distinguish red from green, as there are no L-cones offering a response to contrast with the signals from the M-cones. Missing or faulty M-cones lead to the same deficiency. So-called blue/yellow colour deficiency, caused by faulty or missing S-cones, is extremely rare.

◆ What condition would cause total colour blindness?

◆ If two types of cone are missing, then no colour discrimination could occur.

Total colour blindness occurs extremely rarely.

People with a colour deficiency usually have a problem only in distinguishing shades of red and green, and from a practical point of view cope well with everyday tasks, and may not even be aware of the problem unless they undergo a test. Unfortunately, however, they are precluded from certain professions (Table 3.1) and can often feel discriminated against unfairly. A common test for the presence of red/green colour deficiency is shown in Figure 3.11.

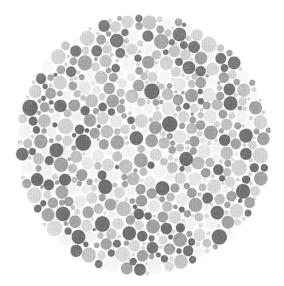

Figure 3.11 An Ishihara test image for red/green colour deficiency, showing the number 73 picked out in green dots on a background of red and yellow dots. If you are colour deficient, you won't be able to distinguish between these colours and so you won't be able to pick out the number from the dots, or you may see a different pattern.

There is currently no effective cure for colour deficiency. Coloured contact lenses and spectacles have been claimed to help some people. The best help that can be given seems to be to increase the red/green distinction (known as red/green contrast) in information to help colour-deficient people, as often they have some residual capacity to discriminate red and green colours.

Summary of Chapter 3

3.1   The three additive primary colours of light – red, green and blue – can be combined in pairs to form the three subtractive primaries – yellow, magenta and cyan. All three additive primaries combine to make white. By extending the range of colours and arranging them to form a colour circle, complementary colours are seen opposite each other: when light of one colour is removed from white light, the colour perceived is the complementary colour.

3.2   Colour is generated by either the absorption or the reflection of light. Objects absorb light of particular wavelengths and the complementary colours reflected are observed by the eye.

3.3   The photoreceptor cells in the retina are rods and cones. Rods outnumber cones 20:1, are more sensitive to light at lower intensities, are distributed over most of the retina except the central foveal region, but they cannot detect colour. Cones, concentrated in the central foveal region, give precise definition to the images seen and detect colour.

3.4   There are three types of cone cells in which the photopigment, retinal, is attached to three different opsin molecules.

3.5   When the retinal molecule absorbs light, it changes shape causing a cascade of events resulting in electrical signals which can be processed and transmitted to the brain via the optic nerve.

3.6   The three different pigments in cones interact with the blue (short wavelengths, S-cones), green (medium wavelengths, M-cones) and red (long wavelengths, L-cones) regions of the visible spectrum.

3.7   The stimulation of the cones in different proportions acts in the same way as the additive primaries, allowing all colours to be perceived.

3.8   Faulty or absent cone cells in a person lead to forms of colour deficiency, most commonly red/green.

Learning outcomes for Chapter 3

After studying this chapter and its associated activities, you should be able to:

LO 3.1   Define and use in context, or recognise definitions and applications of, each of the terms printed in **bold** in the text. (Questions 3.1, 3.2, 3.3 and 3.5)

LO 3.2   Describe how colour is generated either by the absorption or reflection of light, producing complementary colours. (Questions 3.1, 3.2, 3.3 and 3.4)

LO 3.3   At a molecular level describe how the photopigments initiate signals to the brain. (Question 3.4)

LO 3.4   Use trichromacy theory to explain how retinal cone cells discriminate all colours. (Questions 3.2 and 3.4)

LO 3.5   Describe how faulty or absent cone cells leads to forms of colour deficiency. (Question 3.5)

Self-assessment questions for Chapter 3

Question 3.1 (LOs 3.1 and 3. 2)

When an object appears white, which wavelengths of visible light are absorbed and which are reflected?

Question 3.2 (LOs 3.1, 3.2 and 3.4)

Compare and contrast Figures 3.3 and 3.12 and explain why an *unripe* tomato appears green.

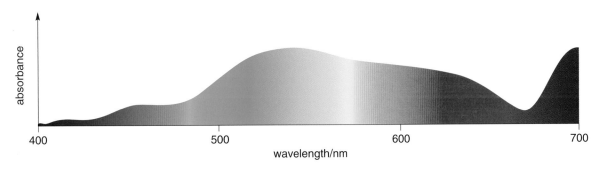

Figure 3.12   Reflection spectrum from the skin of an unripe tomato.

Question 3.3 (LOs 3.1 and 3.2)

Which complementary colour must be absorbed to give each of the following its characteristic colour?

(a) An orange; (b) blood; (c) blue jeans.

Question 3.4 (LOs 3.2, 3.3 and 3.4)

Light of wavelength 590 nm from a sodium street light falls on the eye. Use Figure 3.9 to determine which cones will be stimulated and therefore what colour will be seen by the eye.

Question 3.5 (LOs 3.1 and 3.5)

What colours can and cannot be distinguished if a person has the colour deficiency of missing S-cones?

CHAPTER 4

CORRECTING FOCUSING DEFECTS

4.1 Visual acuity

Focusing defects are a visual impairment in which sight has become blurred. Wearing spectacles can correct for focusing defects and this is a solution adopted in most societies worldwide. This chapter looks in detail at different types of focusing defect, their measurement (through an eye test) and their correction (through spectacle lenses).

Good vision relies on the recognition of objects whether they are close to or far from the observer. This requires good **visual acuity** which is defined as the minimum distance that two lines (or points) must be separated, when viewed at a test distance, to appear as two distinct objects rather than one. Visual acuity is measured by referring to a **Snellen letter chart** (Figure 4.1) which consists of rows of letters of decreasing size. Such measurements are made during an eye test by an optometrist (see Box 4.1).

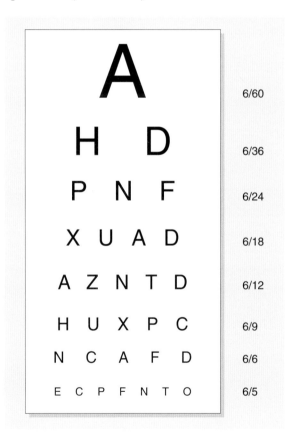

Figure 4.1 A Snellen letter chart. Right-hand numbers indicate the visual acuity required to read successfully the text sizes under test conditions.

Box 4.1 (Enrichment) Eye care professionals

There are several terms for healthcare workers with expertise in eye care. All have different skills and levels of training. In the UK, there are three main categories:

An **ophthalmologist** (op-thal-moll-oh-jist) is a qualified doctor who has specialised in the diagnosis and treatment of eye conditions, and who can perform eye surgery. An **optometrist** (op-tom-met-wrist) is a professional qualified to perform eye tests and record the findings in the form of a spectacle (or contact lens) prescription. An **optician** makes the spectacles or contact lenses from the prescription, and advises on suitable frame or lens choices.

◈ Look at Figure 4.1. Are there any groups of people for whom this would not be a practical test procedure?

◆ The Snellen letter chart relies on the ability to recognise and name the letters. It is therefore not useful when working with very young children or with anyone who is not familiar with the Roman alphabet.

An individual with 'normal' eyesight can read the second smallest row of letters when standing at a distance of 6 metres (20 feet) from the chart. Their visual acuity according to this description is referred to as '6/6' (six : six) or '20/20' (twenty : twenty) vision. The individual's visual acuity can be expressed in terms of how their vision compares with 'normal' vision. This comparison is expressed with the individual's ability as the first number and the 'normal' ability as the second number, thus:

$$\frac{\text{the furthest distance at which the individual being tested can read a line of letters}}{\text{the furthest distance at which a person with 'normal' vision can read the same size letters}}$$

The test was originally devised to be carried out standing 6 metres from the chart so the visual acuity measurement begins with 6; for example, 6/21 would indicate that the individual could see letters clearly at 6 metres which someone with 'normal' sight could see clearly if 21 metres from the chart.

◈ What would a test result of 6/5 mean?

◆ 6/5 means that the individual can see at 6 metres what a person with 'normal' vision can see at 5 metres from the chart.

◈ How would you describe such a person's vision?

◆ They have exceptionally good vision.

◈ Look at Figure 4.1. If an individual could see the letters A; HD; and PNF clearly but not the letters XUAD in the next row, how would their visual acuity be described?

◆ From the right-hand numbers labelling the text size, you can deduce that this person has 6/24 vision. He or she can see at 6 metres what a person with 'normal' vision can see from 24 metres. So this individual's visual acuity is poor.

Very poor visual acuity is the basis for legal definitions of blindness (see Box 4.2).

Box 4.2 (Explanation) Legal definitions of blindness and low vision

In many developed countries, there is educational support and a disability allowance for those whose vision is below an established value. Such legal definitions of *blindness* and *low vision* are based on physical measurements of visual acuity.

In many developed countries, a person is considered **legally blind** when their *corrected* visual acuity (i.e. wearing spectacles) is worse than 6/60.

An individual is considered to have **low vision** when their *corrected* visual acuity is worse than 6/18.

Notice that the definition relates to measurement of the eye's performance after corrective procedures (usually spectacles or surgery) have been applied. It also refers to measurements from the 'better' eye in individuals where vision varies between eyes.

Legal blindness may not mean a total loss of visual perception. Some legally blind individuals may have limited sight, for example in their peripheral vision, which can aid them in everyday life. Alternatively, an individual may have poor vision that restricts their social and work activities, but they may not be classified as legally blind from measurements of visual acuity (e.g. in tunnel vision, see Figure 1.1).

4.2 Common refractive errors

The Snellen letter chart can be used to test for **refractive errors**. These are defects caused by imperfections in the workings of the front region of the eye (the cornea and lens). If you have a refractive error, the refraction process, which re-directs light rays to form the image, does not perform optimally (Figure 4.2). Consequently, a poorly focused image forms on the retina and the world appears blurred. This is because light rays are redirected to form a focused (sharp) image at a point either in front of the retina or behind it (imagining that the retina was transparent and could let light rays through). Refractive errors are the most common types of visual impairment found in the modern world (WHO, 2006).

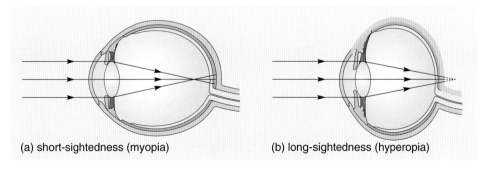

(a) short-sightedness (myopia)   (b) long-sightedness (hyperopia)

Figure 4.2   The point where a sharp image would be formed in the eye, corresponding to where light rays converge in (a) short-sight (myopia); (b) long-sight (hyperopia). Dotted lines show the path that light rays would take if not absorbed by the retina in long-sightedness.

Refractive errors are identified by the optometrist, testing one eye at a time, in case of possible differences between eyes. Working in a darkened room (where the lighting conditions are controlled), the optometrist places lenses over one eye whilst the individual looks at the Snellen letter chart and decides which lens improves vision the most.

◆ Borrow a pair of spectacles from a friend or family member, or if you require spectacles in everyday life, remove them for a moment. Look at a range of objects close to you and far away from you. What do you notice?

◆ This change to your vision makes the world appear blurred or hazy. Objects have lost their sharp edges and fine details.

One observation you may have made was that blurring was particularly apparent from viewing objects *either* far away *or* close up. This is a feature of the two main types of refractive error, myopia and hyperopia, which we will discuss next in this chapter. They cause visual impairment in a manner that varies according to the distance of the object from your eyes.

Myopia

Myopia (also known as short-sightedness or near-sightedness) is the term used to describe the situation where someone is unable to focus clearly on distant objects, although they have no problem with close-up objects (Figure 4.2a).

◆ Study Figure 4.2a and describe where the sharpest image would be formed. What kind of image would be formed on the retina?

◆ The sharpest image would form at a point *in front* of the retina, in the vitreous humour, where the light rays cross. As the retina is not at this position, an unfocused image will be formed on the retina.

This refractive error results from one of two causes. Either the front-to-back distance of the eyeball is too long, or the anatomy at the front of the eye refracts light rays to a greater extent than necessary. In both cases, refracted light rays produce the sharpest image of the world at a point in front of the retina. So retinal cells detect light from an imperfect image, resulting in blurred vision. This focusing defect is often discovered in childhood or early teenage years, as with Rob in Vignette 4.1, where rapid growth of the eye can cause the eyeball to increase disproportionately with the other structures in the eye.

Both genetic and environmental factors contribute to the high incidence of myopia in human populations. Research has shown that two independent factors – a family history of myopia and prolonged **nearwork activity** in childhood – increase an individual's likelihood of developing myopia (Goss, 2000). Nearwork activity involves the eye focusing at close distances for long periods while reading, or viewing computer or television screens.

Vignette 4.1   Myopia in childhood: Rob's story

Rob was a friendly, intelligent child. He was doing well at school. His handwriting was neat and he was especially good at maths. He was very competitive and active. He enjoyed playing football and could run really fast with the ball. However, he was not good at games that involved catching a ball. It amazed him that his brother was so good at catching; Rob just couldn't get himself to the right position fast enough.

Rob was eight when his teacher noticed that, despite having moved closer to the front of the class, Rob screwed up his eyes and 'peered' at the board as though he was having trouble reading it. She decided to talk to his mother.

Rob went with his mother to the optometrist and could not read all the letters on the Snellen letter chart. He managed the first five rows fine but he made a number of mistakes with the sixth row. The optometrist said he had 6/12 vision and was short-sighted as he could not see distant objects clearly. He was prescribed spectacles to wear. Very soon he was learning to play tennis like his brother, which pleased him enormously. However, there were times when wearing spectacles frustrated him such as when walking to school in the rain as water drops would coat the lenses.

Hyperopia

Hyperopia (also known as hypermetropia, long-sightedness or far-sightedness) is the term used to describe the situation where someone is unable to focus clearly on objects that are very close to them. (Figure 4.2b)

⬦ Study the refraction of light rays in Figure 4.2b and describe where the sharpest image would be formed from the ray trace diagram.

◆ The sharpest image would form at a point *behind* the retina (were this possible and light rays could pass through the retina).

Hyperopia results from either the eyeball being too short from front-to-back, or more commonly from incorrect functioning of the cornea and lens at the front of the eye. In both cases, light rays are not refracted sufficiently to form a sharp image at the position of the retina. Vision will therefore be blurred.

4.3   Correcting short- and long-sightedness

To understand how spectacles or contact lenses correct short- and long-sightedness, it is necessary to define the focusing abilities, or *strength*, of a lens.

A lens that forms a sharp image at a large distance is referred to as a *weak* lens, or in scientific terms as a lens with low **optical power**. Optical power is the quantity – measured in the unit dioptres (dye-op-ters) (D) – that an optometrist uses to describe the lens performance. In Activity 2.1, you saw that changing the curvature of a convex lens (by increasing its thickness) changed the focal length.

A thin lens had a long focal length, and formed sharp images a large distance away from the lens. A thick lens had a short focal length and formed sharp images nearer to the lens. This thick lens is referred to commonly as a *powerful* lens, or a lens with a high optical power.

The optical power (in dioptres, D) is the *inverse* of the focal length (in metres). This is written mathematically as

$$\text{optical power (D)} = \frac{1}{\text{focal length (m)}} \tag{4.1}$$

An inverse value is the number obtained by dividing 1 by the respective value. For example, the inverse of $5 = \frac{1}{5} = 0.2$, which you can check with a calculator by pressing

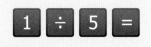

Focal length always uses the unit of metres, despite many convex lenses having focal lengths of only a few centimetres. It is therefore necessary to convert any focal length value in centimetres into metres before calculating the optical power of a lens. Such a conversion gives answers of optical power in the correct unit of dioptres.

◆ Use Equation 4.1 above to calculate the optical power of a convex lens with a 10 cm (centimetre) focal length.

◆ 10 cm is 0.10 m so the optical power in dioptres (D) is the inverse of 0.10, that is, 1 divided by $0.10 = 10$ D.

Because optical power and focal length are inversely related, it is possible to rearrange Equation 4.1 so that you can determine the focal length of a lens if you know its optical power.

$$\text{optical power (D)} = \frac{1}{\text{focal length (m)}} \tag{4.1}$$

which can be rearranged as:

$$\text{focal length (m)} = \frac{1}{\text{optical power (D)}} \tag{4.2}$$

All lens shapes described so far in this book have been convex. Lenses with a *negative* value of optical power (for example -10 D), are called *concave* lenses, and are additionally needed in some spectacles. They are introduced in DVD Activity 4.1.

Activity 4.1   Correcting short- and long-sightedness

Allow about 1 hour. You will need a calculator and some scrap paper.

Activity 4.1 is a multimedia exercise on the DVD associated with this book that builds on your knowledge of lenses from Chapter 2. The properties of **concave** lenses are described and compared with those of convex lenses. Concave lenses have a shape that is thinner at the centre than at the top and bottom extremities. This activity demonstrates with cross-sectional diagrams through the eye how spectacles correct short- and long-sightedness using concave and convex lenses.

Please complete this activity as soon as possible; it will enhance your understanding of the rest of the chapter.

Spectacles place a further lens in front of the cornea and the natural lens inside the eye. The effect of placing several lenses close together is examined in the activity. The combined optical power of two lenses that are close together (called D_{TOTAL}) can be calculated by adding together the optical power of each individual lens (called D_1 and D_2), i.e.

$$D_{TOTAL} = D_1 + D_2 \qquad (4.3)$$

Therefore a convex lens of 30 D (= D_1) and a concave lens of –5 D (= D_2) would produce an overall optical power D_{TOTAL}:

$$D_{TOTAL} = 30 + (-5)$$

$$D_{TOTAL} = 30 - 5$$

$$D_{TOTAL} = 25 \text{ D}$$

This equation is said aloud as 'dee total equals dee-one plus dee-two'.

Adding a negative number is mathematically the same as subtracting that number.

The eyeball of an adult has a diameter of approximately 2 cm (0.02 m). The total focal length of the cornea and lens, for a relaxed eye looking into the distance, must equal this diameter, which is shown in Activity 4.1. So the total optical power, D_{TOTAL}, of an average human eye, when relaxed, can be calculated from:

$$\text{optical power (D)} = \frac{1}{\text{focal length (m)}} = \frac{1}{0.02 \text{ m}} = 50 \text{ D}$$

This value varies between individuals, and also changes during childhood development as the eye grows. So it is a value with little relevance to the *quality* of an individual's vision. On an eye test prescription, the optometrist instead records the optical power (in dioptres) of the lens that best aids vision of the Snellen chart.

Activity 4.1 also shows that a *concave* lens (with a negative optical power) is required to correct short-sightedness, while a *convex* lens (with positive optical power) corrects long-sightedness.

◆ Three friends have the following spectacles prescriptions. Who is (a) long-sighted (b) weakly short-sighted (c) strongly short-sighted?

Johnny: –1.25 D; Sarah: –4.50 D; Pierre: +2.00 D.

◆ (a) Pierre is long-sighted as his prescription has a positive dioptre value. Johnny and Sarah are both short-sighted; (b) Johnny weakly and (c) Sarah strongly. This can be determined by the larger corrective value of her prescription.

4.4 Other refractive errors

Spectacles of a more complex design are required to correct two other common refractive errors.

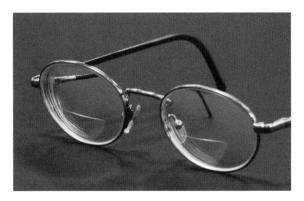

Figure 4.3 Bifocal spectacles for presbyopia. (Source: Roger Courthold)

Presbyopia

Presbyopia (pres-bye-oh-pee-ah) is the term used to describe the decreased ability of the eye lens to accommodate and change optical power. This results from loss of elasticity in the structure of the lens and is a feature that can develop usually beyond the age of 40 (this is described further in Section 6.1). In presbyopia, the lens has hardened and lost some ability to change shape. One consequence for a short-sighted person may be that far away objects still require corrective spectacles, but viewing nearby objects (such as text in a book) now also becomes difficult.

Bifocal lenses are the optometrist's solution (Figure 4.3). These usually have a flat or concave shape (concave to correct for any life-long short-sightedness), but have an additional convex lens attached to the lower portion, in the region of the spectacle lens that one looks through while reading. So when eyes look up to see into the distance, there is correction for any short-sightedness, but when reading and looking down, there is increased optical power to aid reading. Varifocal lenses take this idea a stage further, and use advanced technology to create spectacle lenses with a gradual increase in optical power towards the lower part of the lens.

Astigmatism

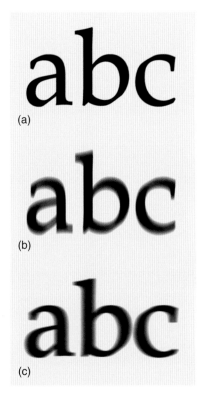

(a)

(b)

(c)

Another type of refractive error results if the cornea is not perfectly symmetrical, with curvature of the cornea in the horizontal direction different from that in the vertical direction. As a result, the cornea is shaped as if slightly compressed or stretched in one direction. This is known as **astigmatism**. In astigmatism, an irregular curvature gives rise to multiple focal points, so a single sharp image does not form on the retina. Thus vision will appear blurred, but this blurring tends to occur predominantly in one direction (vertically or horizontally). A representation of how this affects vision is shown in Figure 4.4. Spectacles can correct for this using specially shaped lenses.

An optometrist makes eye test measurements to prescribe a corrective lens shape and optical power for each eye (usually to the nearest 0.25 D). Measurements are also made to determine the extent of any presbyopia or astigmatism. While spectacle lenses can have complex shapes to correct for any combination of these refractive errors, many people still find spectacle frames restrictive and unsuitable for an active lifestyle or busy job. The next chapter examines two techniques that correct refractive errors without using spectacles.

Figure 4.4 The effects of astigmatism on vision, with blurring in only the orientation where there is incorrect curvature of the cornea. (a) No astigmatism; (b) vertical astigmatism; (c) horizontal astigmatism.

Summary of Chapter 4

4.1 Visual acuity is the ability to perceive a sharply focused image and can be tested using a Snellen letter chart.

4.2 If, even after correction, visual acuity in the better eye is worse than 6/18 it is described as low vision. Anything worse than 6/60 is classified as legally blind in many developed countries.

4.3 The eye forms an image on the retina for objects at different distances by varying the optical power of the lens of the eye.

4.4 Refractive errors result from a poorly focused image on the retina. The sharpest image would form either in front of the retina or (if light rays could pass through it) behind the retina.

4.5 The two main types of refractive error are myopia (short sight) and hyperopia (long sight). These can be corrected by wearing appropriate spectacles to modify the optical power of the eye.

4.6 Myopia and hyperopia cause visual impairment in a manner that varies according to the distance of the object from the eyes.

4.7 The principal focal length and optical power of a lens are determined using light with parallel rays. Such parallel light rays come from objects far away.

4.8 The principal focal length (in metres, m) and optical power (in dioptres, D) are positive in value for convex lenses, and negative for concave lenses.

4.9 The optical power of several lenses close together can be determined by adding together their individual optical powers. This property allows spectacle lenses to correct focusing defects.

4.10 A concave lens can correct for short-sightedness (myopia) and a convex lens for long-sightedness (hyperopia).

4.11 Presbyopia and astigmatism are additional refractive errors which require lenses of complex design for correction.

Learning outcomes for Chapter 4

After studying this chapter and its associated activities, you should be able to:

LO 4.1 Define and use in context, or recognise definitions and applications of, each of the terms printed in **bold** in the text. (Question 4.1)

LO 4.2 Describe how the Snellen letter chart can be used to provide a measure of visual acuity. (Question 4.1)

LO 4.3 Describe the two main types of refractive error, myopia and hyperopia, and their cause in terms of image formation within the eye. (Questions 4.2 and 4.3 and DVD Activity 4.1)

LO 4.4 Calculate focal length and optical power for convex and concave lenses given appropriate lens properties. (Question 4.4 and DVD Activity 4.1)

LO 4.5   Calculate optical powers for a system of more than one lens given individual values of optical power or focal length. (Question 4.5 and DVD Activity 4.1)

LO 4.6   Explain the choice of lens needed to correct long- and short-sightedness. (Question 4.6 and DVD Activity 4.1)

Self-assessment questions for Chapter 4

You also had the opportunity to demonstrate LOs 4.3 to 4.6 by completing Activity 4.1 on the DVD.

Question 4.1 (LOs 4.1 and 4.2)

At the optometrist I am tested with the Snellen letter chart. I can correctly read the text XUAD but not the line below this, and the optometrist says I have 6/18 vision. What does 6/18 vision mean and which of the following statements (a)–(d) best describes my eyesight?

(a) I have myopia.
(b) I have hyperopia.
(c) I have presbyopia.
(d) I have normal vision.

Question 4.2 (LO 4.3)

Myopia leads to objects far away appearing blurred. Does this blurring occur because sharp images form (a) in front of the retina or (b) behind the retina (were this possible and light rays able to pass through the retina)?

Question 4.3 (LO 4.3)

Looking through old wedding photographs, you find a picture that is slightly blurred. The photographer used a tripod, so there was no movement of the camera. Suggest why this blurring occurred.

Question 4.4 (LO 4.4)

An optometrist is examining the left eye of Susan, a 5-year-old girl. When her eye is relaxed, the combined optical power of her cornea and lens is 66 D. What is the overall focal length of the cornea and relaxed lens?

Question 4.5 (LO 4.5)

If the optical power of Susan's left cornea in Question 4.4 was +59 D, what would the optical power of her lens be when it is relaxed?

Question 4.6 (LO 4.6)

If I require concave lenses in my spectacles, am I short- or long-sighted?

CHAPTER 5

CORNEAL SURGERY AND CONTACT LENSES

5.1   Introduction

As you saw in Section 2.4, most of the refraction and focusing of light by the eye takes place at the cornea; the lens simply fine-tunes the focusing. Rather than using spectacles, an alternative method of correcting short- and long-sight is therefore to change the shape of the cornea. This can be done in two ways: the first is to alter the external shape of the cornea by surgery; the second is to cover the cornea directly with a suitably curved piece of plastic – a contact lens. Corneal transplantation is also a future possibility. In this chapter we look at some of the science underlying the first two methods.

5.2   Corneal surgery

Since the 1980s laser eye surgery has become an increasingly popular treatment in the developed world for correcting short- or long-sightedness. Lasers work by reshaping the outer surface of the cornea, and in doing so modify the optical power of the cornea (Figure 5.1). Box 5.1 explains how lasers produce light of sufficient energy to destroy tissue.

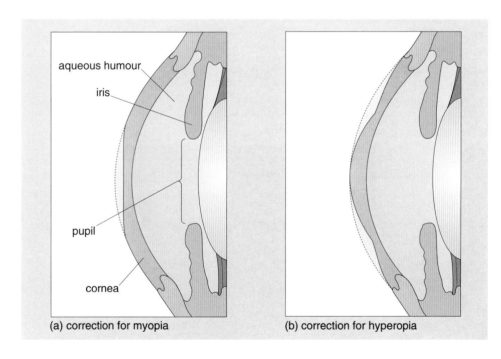

(a) correction for myopia

(b) correction for hyperopia

Figure 5.1   A laser is used to reshape the cornea in order to correct refractive errors. (a) For myopia, a flat profile is produced at the centre of the cornea; (b) for hyperopia, a steep curvature is produced at the centre. Dashed lines indicate the shape of the original cornea.

5.2.1   Laser eye correction – PRK

The original laser technique is known as **PRK**, photorefractive keratectomy (in reference to cutting away or excising part of the cornea to improve refractive errors, using photons). In order to reshape the cornea permanently, the outer layer of protective cells – the corneal epithelial cells – must be removed to allow access to the stroma tissue of the cornea (Section 2.1). Laser reshaping is permanent because the stroma cannot regenerate. In PRK the removal of the epithelial cells is done by chemical or mechanical methods before laser treatment is applied. The epithelial cells subsequently regrow. Nowadays this technique tends to be used only in a small percentage of cases – involving very flat or thin corneas which make the more recent LASIK technique (Section 5.2.2) impractical. As you will see in the next section LASIK (laze-ick) has the advantage of only slightly damaging the epithelial layer, so reducing recovery time and postoperative pain.

Box 5.1 (Enrichment) Lasers and laser safety

A **laser** is a device that produces light of a single wavelength which is transmitted in a narrow powerful beam. Lasers produce light by generating photons through a process known as 'stimulated emission': when a photon passes through a special medium in a laser (often a crystal or a gas), an identical photon is produced which then travels alongside the first photon. By reflecting the light many times through this crystal or gas, many such *photon doublings* occur, resulting in the intense beam of light.

Laser beams can deliver a very large amount of light energy to a very small area, and can damage objects in the beam, such as eyes. Lasers are rated in four classes (I–IV) with Class I being safe for use in all circumstances and Class IV being highly dangerous

to unprotected eyes, even when viewed at a great distance. For laser safety, some operators need to wear special laser goggles that filter out the single wavelength produced by the laser and so prevent the laser light from entering their eyes (Figure 5.2). Without eye protection, the cornea and lens can focus the full energy of the laser onto a very small region of the retina and so burn and destroy the rods and cones there, forming a permanent blind spot area.

Class I lasers are commonly used in supermarkets for scanning barcodes, and Class III lasers in CD players (with a safety interlock incorporated which prevents the laser being viewed). One medical use of Class IV lasers is in surgery to remove or cut tissue.

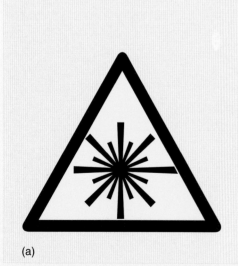

(a)

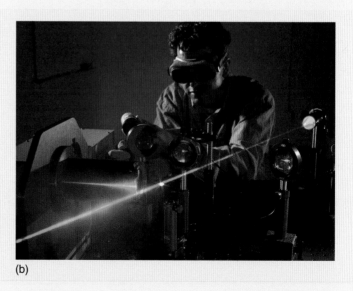

(b)

Figure 5.2 (a) The international hazard symbol for a laser. (b) A research worker using a high-intensity laser source. (Source: David W. Hahn, http://plaza.ufl.edu/dwhahn)

The laser used for PRK or LASIK is a particular kind of laser, an *excimer* (ex-sigh-mer) laser, which produces light in the ultraviolet (UV) region of the electromagnetic spectrum. Ultraviolet light is divided into three bands depending on photon wavelength. UVA (wavelength 400–320 nm) and UVB (320–290 nm) are associated with the harmful effects of sunlight, such as sunburn and skin cancer. UVC (290–180 nm) has the highest photon frequency but cannot penetrate through the Earth's ozone layer in the upper atmosphere, and so is not present in sunlight. The excimer laser produces UVC photons, which can cut through living tissue very precisely, without damaging deeper tissues.

The particular wavelength of the excimer laser (193 nm) is fully absorbed by the cornea of the eye, and cannot pass into the inner eye, so there is no possibility of damage to the retina. The disadvantage is that a UV laser beam cannot be seen by the surgeon, who must use a second very low energy visible 'targeting laser' to align the beam accurately.

◆ Think about photon frequency, rather than wavelength. Does UV have a higher or lower photon wave frequency than visible light? (See Section 2.2.)

◆ UV photons have a *higher* wave frequency than visible light photons.

The energy of a photon can be calculated from its wave frequency, as shown in Box 5.2 overleaf; *photon energy increases in magnitude as photon frequency increases*. UV radiation has a greater frequency than visible light so therefore has greater photon energies. This is important in understanding why UV lasers are used in laser eye surgery.

Photon energies are discussed in another book in this series, *Screening for Breast Cancer* (Parvin, 2007).

The UV photons have sufficient energy to excite the bonding electrons in a molecule to the extent that they can break the chemical bonds and so can damage tissue by breaking apart structural molecules. In laser eye surgery, the energy of one UVC photon in the laser beam breaks one chemical bond at the cornea surface. Treatment is performed by dividing the laser beam into very short pulses that can then be delivered in a controlled manner by the surgeon. Each timed pulse of laser light contains a fixed number of photons, which will in turn break a fixed number of chemical bonds. As the cornea is made up of a uniform matrix of structural molecules, each pulse will break down a constant volume of tissue containing a known number of bonds. Typically, an eye surgery laser with wavelength 193 nm will break down and destroy a 0.25 micrometre (0.25 µm) depth of cornea per pulse. The surgeon applies a predetermined number of pulses to each calculated position in the cornea.

The process of laser eye surgery starts by measuring the thickness of the cornea and then creating a topographic map showing the contours of the surface of the eye using special instrumentation, so that the amount to be removed at each position on the cornea can be calculated.

Box 5.2 (Enrichment) Photon energy and Planck's constant

Figure 5.3 shows the variation of photon frequency and energy across the visible light and lower ultraviolet range of the electromagnetic spectrum.

If E is used to represent the photon energy (measured in joules, J) and f to represent the wave frequency (in hertz, Hz or s^{-1}), then it is found that the energy of a photon is directly proportional to its wave frequency. This relationship can be expressed by the equation:

$$E = h \times f$$

or, as it is often conventional in mathematics to leave out the multiplication signs:

$$E = hf \qquad (5.1)$$

The symbol h represents a constant known as Planck's constant, after Max Planck, a famous German physicist. It has the value 6.626×10^{-34} J s (a *very* small number).

To understand the units of Planck's constant (J s), you need to rearrange Equation 5.1 so that you have h on the left-hand side. You can do this in stages:

First, dividing through Equation 5.1 by f gives:

$$\frac{E}{f} = h \text{ (you must divide both sides of the equation by } f \text{ for everything to remain equal).}$$

Now write the equation with h on the left:

$$h = \frac{E}{f} \qquad (5.2)$$

The units of Planck's constant are thus those of energy (J) divided by the units of frequency (Hz, or s^{-1}), i.e. $\frac{J}{s^{-1}}$ which can be written as J s.

The collagen fibres of the stroma consist of molecules containing mostly C—O, C—H and C—N bonds (chemical bonding is discussed in Section 3.4.2). Note that visible light photons do not have enough energy to break these bonds (Figure 5.3). Lasers used in eye surgery have UV photon energies in excess of these bond energies, and so are able to break the bonds and effectively 'cut' the stroma tissue.

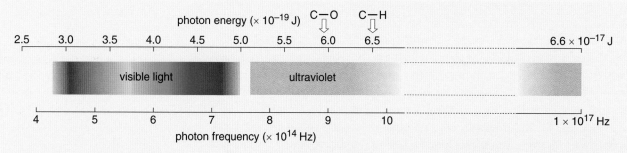

Figure 5.3 Photon frequency and energy in the visible light and lower ultraviolet range. Photon energy is compared with the energy needed to break the chemical bonds C—O and C—H in stroma tissue. The frequency range for ultraviolet extends to 1×10^{17} Hz, which is not shown to scale beyond the C—H bond.

Figure 5.4 shows that by varying removal of tissue at the extreme and central regions, one can change a rectangular block to a convex or concave shape. Figure 5.5 shows the same process applied to the cornea to make the surface less curved, thus increasing the focal length (Section 4.3).

◆ How is the cornea shaped to correct long-sight?

◆ Curvature is increased by removing tissue at the edges, thus increasing the power of the lens and shortening the focal length.

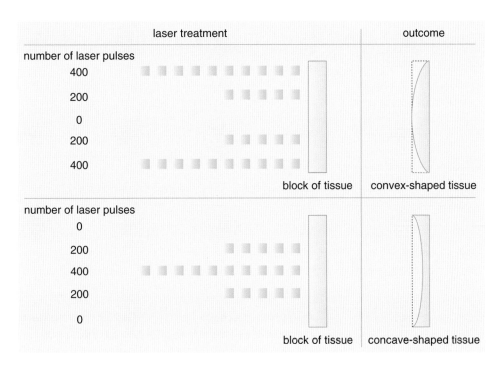

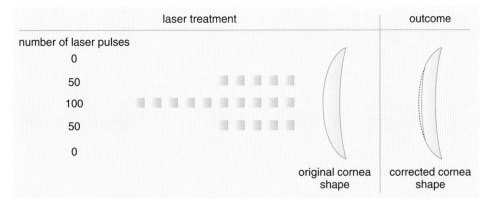

Figure 5.4 How laser treatment could be used to create concave and convex shapes.

Figure 5.5 Applying more pulses at the centre of the cornea reduces the outer curvature and thus the optical power, thus correcting myopia (short-sight).

One problem with this removal of the outer tissue is that the surface of the eye is no longer smooth, leading to haze around bright lights and slight separation of the colours within light. LASIK, the newer laser eye surgery, does not have this disadvantage and is now the most commonly used technique.

5.2.2 Laser eye correction – LASIK

Keratomileusis (ker-at-oh-mil-you-sis) is a medical term meaning the surgical alteration of cornea shape. The process known as **LASIK**, laser-assisted *in situ* keratomileusis, is performed in a single short operation, requiring only a local anaesthetic. A two-stage procedure is performed. Firstly, a flap is cut at the cornea surface and peeled back. Laser treatment then removes corneal tissue *underneath* this flap, so that once the flap is put back, the outer surface of the eye has a new shape but the surface remains smooth. As the flap is returned, very little of the epithelial layer has been traumatised, and the cornea naturally reseals within a few minutes. Now watch the videos in Activity 5.1 describing this procedure.

Activity 5.1   LASIK

Allow 30 minutes

Activity 5.1, in four parts on the DVD associated with this book, will enable you to study the laser eye surgery process. You will watch four videos that illustrate how LASIK is used to correct refractive error in the eye: Activity 5.1a 'Introduction'; Activity 5.1b 'The procedure'; Activity 5.1c 'The laser'; and Activity 5.1d 'The operating theatre'. **Some of the videos show actual eye surgery** and some of you may be uncomfortable viewing surgical procedures. Activity 5.1b shows a 3D animation of the LASIK process in which there is no surgical footage.

There is an option to call up short questions at the end of each video sequence. Once you have thought about them, press the option to reveal answers.

The majority of people who opt for these surgical procedures are very happy with the results, with 6/6 vision or better achieved by over 85% of procedures (Hammond et al., 2005). But of course all surgery carries certain risks such as infection, and a small percentage (3%) of people report ongoing problems such as dry eyes, insufficient correction, poor flap healing and blurred vision or glare.

The next section discusses correcting the shape of the cornea by fitting a contact lens and also looks at the materials that make this possible.

5.3   Contact lenses

The example of contact lenses illustrates how many different science disciplines are vital to advances made in the health sciences. In earlier sections, you have already seen the importance of understanding the physics of optics in correcting sight defects and the chemistry of pigments in colour vision. This section looks at the development of new materials – polymers – for contact lenses.

Contact lenses use their curvature to correct either short- or long-sight. By cancelling out irregularities of the cornea with equal but opposite irregularities of the inner surface of the contact lens, it is also possible to correct astigmatism. The first contact lenses introduced in the late 19th century were made of glass (Figure 5.6) and caused many problems to the wearers. The fundamental problem was the inability of the oxygen in the air to pass through the lens material and get to the surface of the eye. Corneal material is living tissue and carries out the process of **cellular respiration** (where oxygen is used in chemical reactions that provide the cells with energy). Most body tissues are supplied with oxygen by the blood, but the cornea has no blood supply. Instead it gets its oxygen directly from the surrounding atmosphere: the oxygen dissolves in the tears on the surface of the eye and then *diffuses* into the cornea. **Diffusion** is the movement of molecules from regions of high concentration into regions of lower concentration, until there is an even distribution throughout the available volume. If the respiring tissue is starved of oxygen, undesirable effects impair or even destroy corneal function: symptoms include blurred vision, discomfort and a condition called 'red eye'.

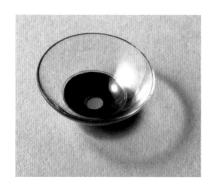

Figure 5.6   An early glass contact lens, c. 1930, made by Myller Söhne Wiesbaden of Germany. (Source: Science Museum/Science Photo Library)

Respiration is discussed in another book in this series (Midgley, 2008).

5.3.1   Hard contact lenses

The first hard plastic lenses were developed in the 1940s and were made from a *polymer* known commonly as Perspex™, known by chemists as PMMA.

Polymers

A **polymer** is a long-chain molecule made up of many repeating units. Each individual repeat unit is formed from a small monomer molecule, usually containing a double bond, and many thousands of units can link together to make the chain.

When polymers are synthesised (usually by heating) the double bond in the monomer breaks and new bonds form with neighbouring monomers. This process repeats until a long chain is formed, shown below for the polymer called polythene.

Table 5.1 shows the structures of the monomers and repeat units of two familiar examples, polythene and Teflon™. It is conventional to enclose the repeat unit in square brackets where the lines indicate the covalent bonds made with the next unit. '*n*' indicates the large number of units joined together to form the polymer. ('*n*' is often used to represent a large number, even colloquially as in 'to the *n*th degree'.)

Table 5.1 Two commonly used polymers.

Common name	Repeat unit	Monomer structure and name
polyethylene or polythene	$-[CH_2-CH_2]_n$	ethene
Teflon	$-[CF_2-CF_2]_n$	tetrafluoroethene

The number of repeat units in a polymer chain varies (for polythene it is 20 000–30 000). Teflon is a very similar polymer structure with the hydrogens replaced by fluorine atoms which confer the well-known 'non-stick' properties.

Polymers can form branched chains, and can also form bonds between chains, a process known as cross-linking; this allows the polymers to form complex networks (Figure 5.7).

A wide range of polymers occur in nature, for example proteins such as collagen. These can be very complex as they consist of very long chains made from monomers called *amino acids*.

For interest, this is the monomer of Perspex (PMMA):

The acronym stands for **poly(methyl 2-methylacrylate)**.

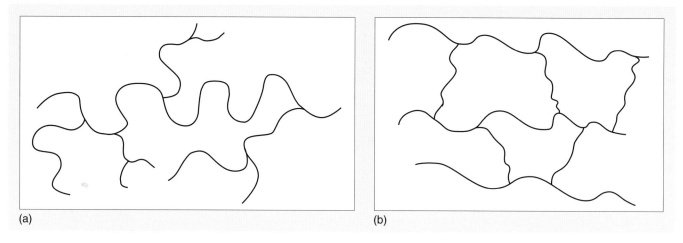

Figure 5.7 (a) A branched chain polymer. (b) A network polymer with cross-linking between chains.

The early Perspex lenses were around 11 mm in diameter, and covered most of the cornea. Almost no oxygen diffused through them, often resulting in sore eyes and temporary distortions of the cornea.

Advances in the development of polymers now allows the production of 'gas permeable' hard lenses that allow unrestricted oxygen diffusion, and offer users round-the-clock wearability.

5.3.2   Soft contact lenses

For many people, hard contact lenses are not an option as they make their eyes very sore. The challenge for chemists has been to find a soft material that does not irritate the eye yet is strong enough to hold its shape as a lens. The solution lay in a material that was more like the cornea itself in structure – a gel (Box 5.3).

The most widely used of all gels in soft contact lens manufacture is PHEMA, a polymer with a complex repeat unit shown below:

$$\left[-CH_2-\underset{\underset{O(CH_2)_2OH}{\overset{\overset{CH_3}{|}}{\underset{|}{C}}}{\overset{|}{\underset{C=O}{|}}}-CH_2-\underset{\underset{O(CH_2)_2OH}{\overset{\overset{CH_3}{|}}{\underset{|}{C}}}{\overset{|}{\underset{C=O}{|}}}-CH_2-\underset{\underset{O(CH_2)_2OH}{\overset{\overset{CH_3}{|}}{\underset{|}{C}}}{\overset{|}{\underset{C=O}{|}}}- \right]_n$$

For interest, PHEMA stands for poly(2-**h**ydrox**y**ethyl **m**eth**a**crylate).

The important thing for you to notice about this structure is that PHEMA contains hydroxyl, $-OH$, groups of atoms: in a hydroxyl group, the oxygen atom again tends to pull rather more than its fair share of the electrons in the bond towards itself, making it slightly more negative, whereas the H atom becomes slightly positive in response.

Box 5.3 (Explanation) What is a gel?

Gels are familiar in everyday life, for example edible jellies (Figure 5.8) made from the animal protein gelatin. Only about 3% of the volume of edible jellies is the natural polymer gelatin, the rest is mainly water. They are made palatable by adding colouring, sweetener, and fruit flavours. Gels are also found in the human body; for example the vitreous humour that fills the interior of the eye, and the synovial fluid that lubricates joints.

Why can gels hold so much water? Some atoms are better at attracting electrons to themselves than others and oxygen is one of these, it is said to be **electronegative**. In the water molecule, H—O—H, the oxygen atom tends to pull more of the negatively charged electrons in the bonds towards itself, making it slightly negative, whereas the H atoms become slightly positive as a result. The drift of negatively charged electrons towards the more electronegative element is shown by writing over the oxygen a *partial* negative charge, $\delta-$ (delta-minus), and over the hydrogen atom, a partial positive charge, $\delta+$ (delta-plus):

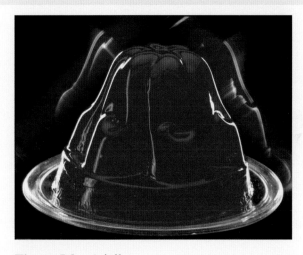

Figure 5.8 A jelly.

The Greek lower-case delta, δ, is conventionally used throughout maths and science to represent a small or partial quantity.

$$\overset{\delta+}{H}-\overset{\delta-}{O}-\overset{\delta+}{H}$$

where the $\delta-$ indicates that the bonding electrons spend more time near the oxygen nucleus and less time near the hydrogen nucleus ($\delta+$).

One of the effects of this separation of charge within a molecule is that neighbouring molecules can form weak bonds with each other. (Weak bonds tend to be long, whereas strong bonds are short.) This happens particularly strongly in water, where the $H^{\delta+}$ of one molecule is attracted to the $O^{\delta-}$ of a neighbouring molecule, and is known as **hydrogen bonding** (Figure 5.9).

A gel is intermediate between a solid and a liquid, and consists of polymers that are cross-linked to make a tangled porous network, together with a liquid, usually water. The water molecules fill the pores in the network, making weak hydrogen bonds with the polymer and with each other, and thus prevent the polymer network from collapsing.

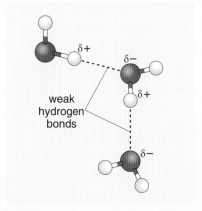

Figure 5.9 Hydrogen bonding between water molecules; the longer, weaker hydrogen bonds are shown dotted. (O red, H white).

Hydrogen-bonding is discussed in another book in this series, *Alcohol and Human Health* (Smart, 2007).

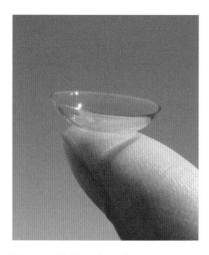

Figure 5.10 A soft contact lens after hydration. (Source: Jane Pang/istockphoto)

◆ Would you expect PHEMA to undergo hydrogen bonding with water molecules?

◆ Yes, the hydroxyl, —OH, groups can hydrogen-bond with the water molecules.

When this polymer is manufactured (see Activity 5.2), a three-dimensional network is obtained that swells in water as the water molecules become organised in the pores to give a rigid gel, which does not dissolve in water. The polymer network can absorb about 40% by mass of water. The ability of the gel to take up a large quantity of water is very desirable for contact lenses because oxygen can dissolve in this trapped water and thus diffuse *through* the contact lens to the cornea. The more the lens resembles a droplet of water, the better the compatibility with the eye. The gel network is there simply to maintain the shape and thus the optical properties (Figure 5.10).

Many people prefer the look of contact lenses to wearing spectacles; they are also comfortable for most people, and make sporting activities easier. More than 70% of contact-lens users now wear soft lenses in preference to hard, but even these new materials are not without problems:

- They are not 100% oxygen permeable, and so soft lenses cannot be worn all day.

- The cornea produces proteins that are absorbed by the gel water; this leads to cleaning and sterilisation problems.

Scientists continue researching to find gel systems that can overcome all these problems. The production and development of contact lenses is covered further in the optional Activity 5.2.

Activity 5.2   A glance at polymers

Allow 20 minutes

This video on the DVD associated with this book, covers the development and manufacture of soft contact lenses, visiting a research laboratory and a factory. It illustrates how disciplines other than medicine and biology – chemistry, physics, and engineering – all contribute richly to health sciences, and shows that continuing research is necessary to keep improving the technologies to correct visual impairments.

Summary of Chapter 5

5.1 Lasers produce narrow beams of intense light in which all the photons have the same wavelength.

5.2 Ultraviolet (UV) lasers are used in laser eye surgery as UVC light cannot penetrate through the cornea into the eye and so there is no risk of damaging the retina.

5.3 UVC photons break chemical bonds and each laser pulse destroys a small depth of corneal tissue.

5.4 Varying the number of pulses at each position can 'machine' a new surface geometry to the cornea enabling the eye to form a sharp image on the retina.

5.5 The first contact lenses, made of glass or the polymer Perspex, prevented oxygen diffusion to the cornea, causing discomfort and blurred vision.

5.6 Polymers are long-chain molecules made from small repeating units (monomers).

5.7 The polymers developed for 'hard' contact lenses allow unrestricted oxygen diffusion.

5.8 'Soft' contact lenses are made from polymeric gels.

5.9 The polymers forming a gel contain electronegative oxygen atoms that form hydrogen bonds with water.

Learning outcomes for Chapter 5

After studying this chapter and its associated activities, you should be able to:

LO 5.1 Define and use in context, or recognise definitions and applications of, each of the terms printed in **bold** in the text. (Questions 5.1 and 5.3)

LO 5.2 Describe the underlying process that occurs in the laser interaction with the molecules which make up the corneal tissues. (Questions 5.1 and 5.2)

LO 5.3 Describe the structure of polymer chains in terms of repeating small chemical units. (Question 5.3)

LO 5.4 Describe the difference between covalent bonding within a polymer chain and the weak hydrogen-bonding to water molecules in gels used to make soft contact lenses which thus support oxygen diffusion. (Question 5.3)

Self-assessment questions for Chapter 5

Question 5.1 (LOs 5.1 and 5.2)

To correct short-sightedness with LASIK treatment, the outer curvature of the cornea must be reduced. Looking at Figure 5.5, how can the laser eye surgeon achieve this?

Question 5.2 (LO 5.2)

Calculate how much depth of cornea, in centimetres, is removed by (a) 100 laser pulses and (b) 20 laser pulses, assuming removal of 0.25 micrometre (or 0.25×10^{-6} m) per pulse.

Question 5.3 (LOs 5.1, 5.3 and 5.4)

The PHEMA polymer forms hydrogen bonds with water. Describe the two types of O—H bond that are present in this structure (Figure 5.9), and say which is the stronger and which the longer.

CHAPTER 6

CHRONIC CONDITIONS THAT CAUSE SIGHT LOSS

You have thus far only studied shortcomings in the apparatus that focuses light onto the retina of the eye. There are, however, ways in which visual impairments can be acquired throughout life, either as a result of progressive structural changes to the eye or as a consequence of repeated eye infections. Structural changes are more prevalent in older people but can also occur in young people, particularly following accidents; children and women seem to be particularly susceptible to eye infections. In this final chapter, you will be studying some chronic conditions that are a major cause of sight loss, cures (where available) and preventative measures.

6.1   Cataract

Cataract is a condition that affects the lens. The lens of the eye is enclosed in a capsule made from a protein called collagen (Figure 6.1). The lens has no blood vessels.

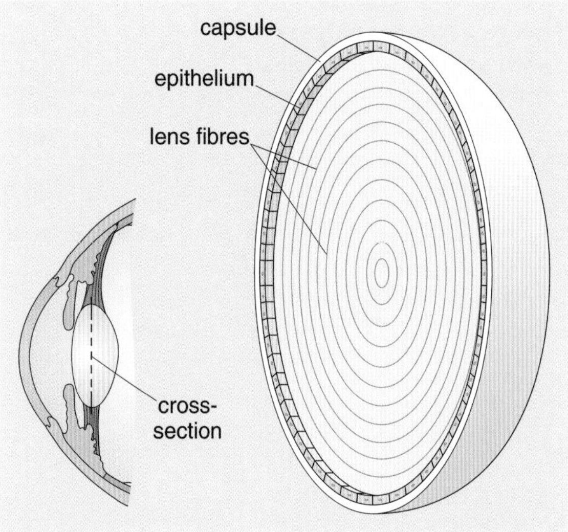

◈   What is the function of the lens?

◆   The lens helps to focus light onto the retina of the eye (Section 2.4).

◈   Why would blood vessels within the lens tissue create a problem?

◆   The lens would not be perfectly transparent so light could not pass through freely.

Figure 6.1   Diagram of a lens showing how an outer protein capsule surrounds the epithelial cell layer.

The lens cells and the proteins within them are very precisely arranged so that light passes through them without being deflected. The outermost cell layer of the lens is formed of epithelial cells (Figure 6.1). As there is no blood supply, the lens epithelial cells have a very low level of metabolic activity. Oxygen and nutrients, such as glucose, are able to diffuse into these cells from the surrounding fluids, but only very slowly. Thus, very slowly, these epithelial cells make new lens cells. Over a lifetime, the lens gradually becomes thicker and less flexible as mature lens cells accumulate.

◈   What is the functional consequence of changing the shape and reducing the flexibility of the lens?

◆   It becomes more difficult to adjust focus (accommodate) and to form a clear image. The individual is said to have presbyopia (see Section 4.4).

A mature lens cell is called a lens fibre (Figure 6.1). It is essentially a sack containing a high proportion of proteins called crystallins in a gel (see Box 5.3). The lens cells make these proteins following 'instructions' from the genetic

Metabolic activity describes all the chemical processes that occur in cells.

material contained in the nucleus of the cell. After making crystallins the lens cells mature by getting rid of the rest of their internal structures, including the nucleus, which means that they can no longer make any more proteins.

The crystallins are therefore unusual in that they are not constantly being broken down and reconstituted by the lens cells (as happens with most body proteins); therefore they must last for life. The disadvantage of this is that they tend to deteriorate over time and cannot be replaced. In fact, from about 40 years old onward the lens may start to cloud (as shown earlier, Figure 1.2) due to this deterioration.

There are a variety of events and substances that accelerate the deterioration of proteins; these include:

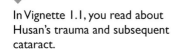

In Chapter 1 and in another book of this series (Midgley, 2008) the connection was made between smoke from unventilated indoor fires and cataract formation.

- heat
- ultraviolet (UVA and UVB) light
- smoke (from fires or from tobacco)
- chemicals (toxins, alcohol)
- trauma
- ionising radiation (X-rays).

Some of these hazards are unavoidable; for example, exposure to daylight includes exposure to UVA and UVB ultraviolet light. However, precautions such as wearing high-quality sunglasses in bright light can reduce the risks.

In Vignette 1.1, you read about Husan's trauma and subsequent cataract.

Most people have heard of cataracts and are aware that they impair sight. Age-related cataracts are so common that it would be unusual not to have an older family member who has had a cataract. But the good news is that cataracts can be treated, so that they need not be a cause of blindness. In the USA, 2 million cataract operations are carried out every year and cataract surgery is the most frequent surgical procedure in many high-income countries. (OECD, 2005). The risk of developing an age-related cataract begins around age 40 years and figures from the USA suggest that half of 80-year-olds either have cataracts or have had cataract surgery.

Nevertheless, age-related cataract is still a major cause of blindness worldwide, affecting 18 million people.

◆ What proportion (or percentage) of world blindness does this represent? (See Figure 6.2.)

◆ This represents almost half (about 48%) of world blindness.

If you are reading this in a high-income country, you may be initially puzzled and alarmed by this statistic. You are probably aware that cataract operations can restore sight and may now be wondering whether these operations are effective. The answer is that over 90% of cataract operations do restore sight.

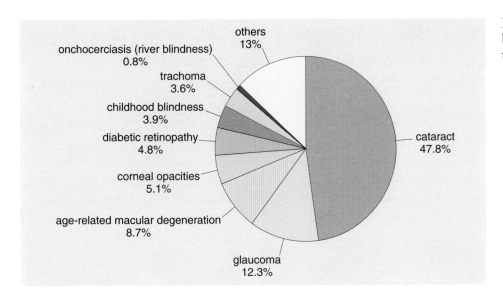

Figure 6.2 Global causes of blindness as a percentage of total blindness in 2002.

The actual operation is very straightforward (as you will see in Activity 6.1). It is usually performed under local anaesthetic, so although the patient feels nothing they can hear and therefore be told what is happening. It takes only about 10 minutes for the surgeon to remove the clouded lens from within the collagen capsule – which in itself is often enough to improve sight significantly.

◆ Can you explain why?

◆ Because most of the focusing is done by the cornea, light can penetrate the eye once the lens has been removed, and can still be focused on the retina.

In most high-income countries, a slightly longer operation is performed in which the clouded lens is replaced by a clear plastic one. The incision is so small that often it is not necessary to put in any stitches and the cut will heal rapidly. The eye will be kept bandaged for at least 24 hours to keep it from becoming infected. In 98% of cases there are no complications and over 90% of patients report that their sight is restored through this operation.

However, while cataract surgery does restore sight, there remains a disadvantage in that overall visual performance is less than before the cataract developed. This is because the new plastic lens cannot accommodate – or change optical power – and so focusing on objects at different distances is harder, particularly if both eyes have had surgery. It is usual for cataract patients to require spectacles for the rest of their lives after surgery – one pair for close reading and another for distance viewing, or alternatively bifocal or varifocal spectacles (see Section 4.4).

In summary, age-related cataract causes almost half of world blindness yet it can be treated successfully by surgery. Reading Vignette 6.1 overleaf (taken from a WHO website) will give you some ideas as to why not everyone with cataract receives treatment.

Vignette 6.1 Treating cataract in rural India: Kuzhanthiammal's story

Two years ago, when she was 65 years old, Kuzhanthiammal began to worry when a white film started to cloud one of her eyes. Her sight rapidly deteriorated, making it hard to work on her land and take care of her family. The nearest hospital was too far away and too expensive to visit.

Soon after her symptoms appeared, Kuzhanthiammal heard that a mobile diagnostic eye clinic was visiting a nearby village. The clinic is run by the Aravind Eye Hospital in Madurai, India, to reach people living in remote, rural villages. Kuzhanthiammal went to the clinic, and within a few minutes, she was diagnosed with cataract (Figure 6.3).

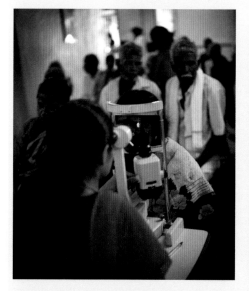
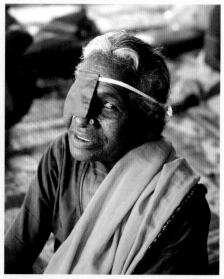

Figure 6.3 The Indian eye clinic. (Source: WHO/Chris de Bode)

Figure 6.4 Kuzhanthiammal after her operation. (Source: WHO/Chris de Bode)

The clinic staff registered Kuzhanthiammal for free cataract surgery the following week at the hospital. The programme also covered transportation costs. 'A bus picked me up with seven other people and drove us to the hospital,' she says.

Around 70% of patients at the hospital receive free eye surgery and follow-up care. They are subsidised by the 30% who are able to pay for their medical care.

Now 67 years old, Kuzhanthiammal successfully underwent surgery on her other eye a few months ago. 'The operation was over so quickly. It's a miracle – it's like waking up with your problems gone.'

◆ From this vignette suggest two reasons why cataract surgery is not available for everyone in the world who needs it.

◆ The vignette indicated two potential problems for Kuzhanthiammal: cost, and distance to appropriate facilities.

In India it is estimated that around 9 million people may already be blind as a consequence of untreated cataract (Venkata et al., 2005). In the last decade of the 20th century, India doubled the number of cataract surgical operations to around 3 million per year (or 300 per 100 000 population); but with an annual incidence of new cases at around 3.8 million people, the backlog of untreated cases keeps growing each year. By comparison, Figure 6.5 shows the number of cataract surgeries per 100 000 population in several OECD countries, i.e. countries belonging to the Organisation for Economic Cooperation and Development, a grouping of 30 democratic industrialised countries from North America, Europe and the Pacific Rim.

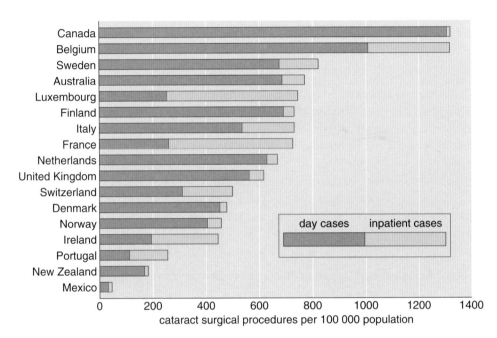

Figure 6.5 Number of cataract surgeries, inpatient and day cases, per 100 000 population in several OECD countries in 2003 or nearest available date. (Day case: patient leaves hospital on the same day as the surgery; inpatient case: patient remains in hospital at least overnight and sometimes for several days after the operation.) (Source: OECD, 2005)

◆ Describe the most striking features of this bar chart.

◆ There is tremendous variation in the number of cases treated per 100 000 population. There is also considerable variation in the proportion of cases where the patient does not remain at the hospital (the day cases). In Canada a tiny minority remain as inpatients, whereas in Luxembourg over half are treated as inpatients.

The amount of time that the patient spends in hospital will affect the cost of the procedure and also the number of people who can be treated. The charity Sightsavers International estimated in 2007 that they could provide a cataract operation for a child for £27 (as in Husan's story in Vignette 1.1).

Despite this relatively low cost, as has been previously noted, cataract is responsible for 48% of global blindness. It is only in the most affluent countries that it is not the number one cause of blindness.

6.2 Glaucoma

Glaucoma is the term used to describe damage to the optic nerve that has been caused, in most cases, by the build-up of pressure within the eyeball (i.e. there

intra from the Greek meaning 'within', *ocular* meaning 'of the eye'.

is an increase in *intraocular* pressure). Why this build-up of pressure causes neurons to die is not really understood. Indeed, some people exhibit optic nerve damage even though their eye pressure is within the normal range for healthy eyes. Their glaucoma is described as *low-tension glaucoma* where low-tension means low pressure.

Some eye specialists believe that people with low-tension glaucoma have super-sensitive neurons within the optic nerve. As is often the case in biology – and in medicine – the connection between cause and effect can be a bit uncertain. Depending on which source of information you consult, you will find that the reason proposed for the optic nerve damage is either that the pressure damages the retinal artery, thereby impairing the supply of oxygen and nutrients to the retina, or that the pressure directly damages the delicate axons of neurons in the optic nerve. Probably there is truth in both of these explanations and maybe different factors are of greater or lesser importance in different people.

What is certain is that when nerve damage has occurred, it cannot be reversed. As some people have glaucoma despite having apparently 'normal' intraocular pressure, it should not surprise you to hear that some people with high intraocular pressure do not have glaucoma. Because of this variability it is important to spot *changes* that may be early danger signs, such as intraocular pressure increasing between one routine eye test and the next. There are other checks on eye health that seek to expose early signs of glaucoma and can be used for anyone who is at particular risk of acquiring the condition, such as anyone with a family history of glaucoma and older people in general. Other groups at risk will be identified as the different types of glaucoma are described.

In order to understand the different types of glaucoma, you need to know how normal eye pressure is maintained. Look back at Figure 2.3 (Section 2.1). The eye has two fluid-filled chambers or cavities. Behind the lens is the vitreous cavity and between the lens and the cornea is a second cavity that is incompletely divided into two areas by the iris. The fluids in all of these spaces are transparent.

◆ Why is it important that these spaces contain transparent fluids?

◆ Light must travel through these spaces without being absorbed to enable a clear image to be formed on the retina at the back of the eye.

The content of the vitreous cavity, known as the *vitreous humour*, is 99% salty water but there are proteins dissolved in the water, giving it a thick consistency.

◆ The vitreous humour is a gel. Describe the chemical composition you would expect it to have. (Think back to Box 5.3.)

◆ The proteins are polymers that are cross-linked to make a tangled porous network. The water molecules fill the pores in the polymer network and the whole structure is held together with weak hydrogen bonds.

The pressure exerted by this gel helps to keep the shape of the eyeball, by pressing gently against the retina.

In the cavity in front of the lens is a fluid called the *aqueous humour*. It is secreted from small blood vessels known as capillaries. A continuous supply of aqueous humour is required by the lens to provide oxygen and nutrients because the lens does not have its own blood supply (as described in Section 6.1). The aqueous humour also supplies nutrients to the cornea.

◆ How does the cornea obtain oxygen?

◆ The cornea obtains oxygen from the air: the oxygen diffuses into the tear fluid and from there into the corneal tissues (Section 5.2).

As aqueous humour is being continuously secreted, there would be a build-up of pressure within this closed space unless fluid is removed at the same rate as it is secreted. In fact, it drains into veins in the eye after passing through *trabeculae* (trab-eck-you-lee), tissue that acts like a filter or sieve, as shown in Figure 6.6.

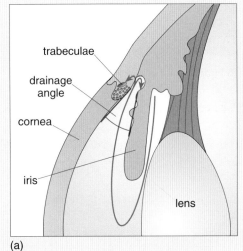
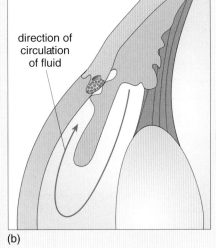

(a)   (b)

Figure 6.6 Diagrammatic cross-section of the front of the eye to show (a) the circulation of aqueous humour (long arrow) and (b) how a blockage can occur when the iris lies too close to the cornea.

The trabeculae fill the space where the cornea and the iris meet. If you look at Figure 6.6a you can see that the iris and cornea meet at an angle, known as the **drainage angle**. If this space becomes blocked, the fluid cannot drain away efficiently, so the intraocular pressure rises and the result is glaucoma.

Obviously this system usually works perfectly. The 'drain' is kept clean by the action of phagocytic (fag-oh-sit-ic) cells found on the surface of the trabeculae. However, particularly with increasing age or as a consequence of an inflammatory reaction, the 'drain' can get silted up. This results in increased pressure within the enclosed space. Increased pressure on the drainage angle will push the aqueous humour through the 'drain' and a new balance between inflow and outflow can be achieved.

Phagocytosis ('fag-oh-sigh-toh-sis') means 'cell-eating' and is derived from the Greek *phaein* meaning to eat and *cyte* meaning cell – note 'cyte' is frequently used in biology, as in *cytosol* and leuko*cyte* (white blood cell).

So with a slight increase in intraocular pressure, outflow and inflow are kept in balance. Thus the onset of this most common form of glaucoma, called **open-angle glaucoma** can be very gradual; a slow, insidious increase in intraocular pressure that can damage the optic nerve. It is a chronic condition, occurring when fluid drains away too slowly and intraocular pressure gradually increases. Initially vision is not impaired and there is no pain. Subsequent deterioration in vision can be so gradual that it too goes unnoticed. This is because, although as axons die and no signal is sent from the parts of the visual field from which information would normally be supplied, nevertheless the brain 'fills in' the missing parts of the 'jigsaw'. For example, we all have a blind spot in our field of view where the optic nerve leaves the eyeball, because there are no photoreceptors (rods and cones) there (Figure 2.3). No-one reports that they are aware of this 'hole' in their visual field. Remember that you performed an experiment to show that you do have this blind spot (see Activity 2.3).

A less common type of glaucoma, but one that can have a rapid onset, is **closed-angle glaucoma** (also known as narrow-angle glaucoma). This condition occurs when the drainage angle (the gap between the cornea and the iris) decreases and the aqueous fluid can no longer drain away efficiently (Figure 6.6b). In a third of cases, the individual is made aware of its presence by an acute episode. The blockage of the drainage angle means that the intraocular pressure increases rapidly. This is accompanied by sudden pain, headache and nausea with blurred vision and/or rainbow-coloured halos around light. Medical attention is needed immediately to reduce eye pressure and prevent further damage to the optic nerve. Examination of the drainage angle when eyes are tested will reveal if the iris and cornea are too close to one another making the eyes prone to this condition. Asians, particularly Chinese people, are peculiarly susceptible to closed-angle glaucoma. (Africans are the ethnic group most susceptible to open-angle glaucoma.)

> An acute episode has a sudden, often dramatic onset.

Glaucoma takes its place on the WHO Vision 2020 priority eye diseases list because of its prevalence. Worldwide there are 4.5 million people with glaucoma.

◆ Looking at Figure 6.2, what position does glaucoma occupy in terms of its contribution to world blindness?

◆ It is second only to cataract in contributing to the burden of blindness globally. In 2002 it accounted for 12% of world blindness.

In the UK glaucoma is responsible for around 8% of blindness despite the fact that there are facilities to detect glaucoma and treatments to prevent it from progressing to cause sight loss. The RNIB has embarked upon an 'Open your Eyes' campaign to publicise the causes of avoidable blindness and urge people to have regular eye tests with the aim of supporting the WHO Vision 2020 initiative to eradicate preventable blindness.

◆ At the asymptomatic stage, how do you suppose an ophthalmologist would test for glaucoma?

◆ Potentially glaucoma could be identified by:

- measuring intraocular pressure
- examining the drainage angle
- examining the state of the optic nerve
- testing to see whether any visual loss had occurred.

It is possible to do all of these things in a full eye test and so it is important to carry out full eye tests for anyone who is identified as being particularly at risk.

◈ What do you suppose would place a person at particular risk of glaucoma?

◆ Important risk factors include:

- age
- ethnicity
- raised intraocular pressure
- genetic predisposition (other family members with glaucoma).

It is not known why glaucoma becomes more prevalent with age, but it may be just part of the general deterioration of functioning that comes with advancing years. In developed countries, the incidence rises from about 2% of the population who are over 40 years of age to around 8% of over 70-year-olds.

In addition to ethnic and genetic predisposition to glaucoma, there is an association with myopia, particularly where myopia is caused by an eyeball with a long front-to-back distance.

Eye infections or injury that could lead to increased 'debris' in the aqueous humour are risk factors, as are any circulatory problems that might result in inefficient drainage.

Although there is no known treatment to prevent the onset of glaucoma, there are treatments available to stop it causing blindness. Most people can be treated for glaucoma using a range of drugs that aim to reduce pressure by either decreasing the secretion of aqueous humour or increasing the rate of drainage. The drugs are given as eye drops, self-administered daily. Unfortunately these drops are not precise in their ability to target the affected area, and that area only. This means that the drops can have other effects (side-effects), such as stinging eyes, focusing difficulties and headaches, that are unpleasant and that can result in non compliance (i.e. patients not using their drops). If the intraocular pressure cannot be lowered using medication then surgery to open up the drainage angle is an option.

Glaucoma can be arrested if diagnosed early enough. Unfortunately glaucoma often goes undiagnosed, even in developed countries, because people do not avail themselves of regular eye tests. For example, a report from the RNIB (2005) estimated that there were a quarter of a million people in the UK at risk of losing their sight because of undiagnosed glaucoma. Because glaucoma can develop slowly and without symptoms or pain it is often called the 'silent thief of sight'.

6.3 Age-related macular degeneration (AMD)

There are a number of conditions that can damage the retina and hence impair vision. The most important in terms of the number of people affected worldwide is **age-related macular degeneration (AMD)**. Globally it is number three as a cause of blindness, accounting for 8.7% of blindness. In the developed world it is the leading cause of blindness, accounting for 50% of blindness and affecting about 1.5 million people.

◈ Of the 37 million blind people worldwide how many are affected by AMD?

◆ Around 3 million people (8.7% of the 37 million blind people).

AMD is the leading cause of blindness in the *developed* world because the condition is age-related and the number of people who live to an old age is greater in the developed than it is in the developing world. Cataract is also age-related and is at the global level a more common condition than AMD (Figure 6.2). Yet it accounts for fewer cases of blindness in the developed world. This reflects the fact that damage to the retina (AMD) is more difficult to treat than clouding of the lens (cataract).

◆ What is the function of the retina?

◆ The photoreceptors of the retina convert light signals into electrical signals. Other retinal cells process and organise these signals into different information streams; for example, information about movement goes to a different part of the brain from information about colour (Box 2.6).

Figure 2.16b showed that light must pass through several layers of cells before it stimulates the photoreceptors.

◆ Figure 2.16b shows the two types of photoreceptors: rods and cones. How do they differ in their functions?

◆ The cones are the least sensitive to light but they mediate colour vision. Rods are very sensitive to light but do not mediate colour vision (Section 2.5).

To enable them to register tiny amounts of light, the rods have a greatly expanded 'working' surface consisting of discs that contain photosensitive pigments (the visual pigments) that react to the photons of light (Figure 2.16c). About 10% of these discs are renewed daily and cells in the retinal pigment epithelium (RPE) 'scavenge' these old discs by phagocytosis. (Cones also renew their visual pigments but much more slowly.)

Rods outnumber cones by about 20:1. However, at the optical axis of the eye (see Figure 2.3) is an area where cones predominate.

◆ What does this area look like?

◆ There is a yellow spot on the retina called the macula lutea at the centre of which is a depression called the fovea (Figure 3.7b).

The colour comes from a yellow pigment called lutein that is present in the axons of neurons in this area. Since light passing to this area of the retina must pass through this region before reaching the cones, the macula lutea acts as a filter.

◆ What colour light will yellow pigments absorb?

◆ They screen out the high-energy purple-blue wavelengths (Figure 3.4).

The transparent lens of the eye also acts as a filter, cutting out the wavelengths below 390 nm. The two filters together screen this part of the retina from potentially damaging UVA and UVB ultraviolet radiation. Nevertheless, damage to the retina can occur. As its name suggests, AMD is a degenerative disease of the retina, though it is not necessarily caused by sunlight. Smoking, a poor diet and a genetic predisposition to AMD are also implicated in the development of this condition.

In AMD the initial degeneration is in the retinal pigmented epithelium (RPE). These cells lose their pigment and atrophy (waste away). As these cells are lost, the phagocytic role of the RPE is reduced and discarded material from the rods and cones may instead start to accumulate locally. In turn, this causes deterioration of the blood vessels of the retina, and then the cells of the retina, including the rods and cones, start to die because their waste products are not being removed fast enough and their supply of nutrients and oxygen is inadequate.

In most cases, the progress of the disease is slow and central vision is lost very gradually allowing low-vision aids to be used. It is rare for AMD to cause total blindness; peripheral vision usually remains. Around 90% of people with AMD have **dry AMD** (as just described) but with some people, this progresses to **wet AMD** when blood vessels from the choroid grow into the macular area. The growth of new vessels is a response to the deterioration of the existing system. Unfortunately the new vessels are invariably weak and start to leak. Leakage of blood into the macula distorts the image or may even obscure it completely. Wet AMD can be treated by sealing off the blood vessels using laser surgery (see Section 6.4) but this must be carried out at an early stage of the disease before scarring of the retinal tissue has caused irreversible damage. A procedure called PDT (photodynamic therapy) uses a light-sensitive dye injected into the bloodstream to locate the vessels that are growing in the wrong place. A more suitable treatment for most cases of wet AMD is the use of anti-VEGF drugs. These drugs block the activity of the protein VEGF (vascular endothelial growth factor) that helps new blood vessels to form. Again, treatment – which involves injections into the eye – must be given at an early stage of the disease.

There is no pain associated with AMD and the condition can only be detected by an eye examination, usually before any symptoms have been experienced. The retina is examined during routine eye examinations at the optician. Unfortunately there is currently no cure for AMD but its progress may be slowed (as above) and some lifestyle changes may be helpful. For example, it is advisable to give up smoking as it is the only known avoidable risk factor that has been established (Thornton et al., 2005).

Wearing high-quality sunglasses to protect the eyes from UVA and UVB radiation from the sun is also recommended.

Finally, some ophthalmologists recommend dietary supplements to slow the progress of the disease. This is based on some studies that suggest that lutein intake affects the macular pigmentation of the eye. Lutein is present in green leafy vegetables such as spinach.

Overall, wet AMD is responsible for more cases of blindness than dry AMD, despite being the less common condition. As the ageing population increases and AMD becomes more prevalent, increasing research effort is going into understanding its causes and into searching for ways to repair damaged retinas (Box 6.1).

Box 6.1 (Enrichment) Retinal repair

The loss of photoreceptor cells (rods and cones) causes irreversible impairment of vision in many diseases that affect the retina (for example, age-related macular degeneration and diabetes). One of the main reasons is that photoreceptor cells are formed early in life and are not replaced if they become damaged later on. Like many other cells of the nervous system, these highly specialised cells cannot replicate themselves and are initially formed from other cells (stem cells) during development.

Stem cells are discussed in another book in this series, *Trauma, Repair and Recovery* (Phillips, 2008). Stem cells are special cells that can divide to produce daughter cells that can become a selection of different cell types.

Scientists have worked for many years to find a way to replace damaged photoreceptor cells in adults. A number of approaches have been tried, the most promising of which currently (2007) is to isolate the stem cells that eventually turn into photoreceptor cells. In 2006 scientists in the UK made a breakthrough when they took cells from one-day-old mice and used them successfully to replace damaged photoreceptor cells in adult mice (MacLaren et al., 2006). The key to the success of this technique was that rather than use stem cells derived from the brain or the retina that have the ability to become a variety of *different* cell types, this team used cells at a later developmental stage which were already destined to become photoreceptor cells. These cells, known as *precursors*, are one of the intermediate cell types in the sequence between stem cells and the final photoreceptor cells. They have the advantage of being able to divide to produce more precursor cells (unlike the final photoreceptor cells) but can also integrate with damaged adult retinas to form new photoreceptor cells (Figure 6.7). These new photoreceptor cells made connections with the neuronal networks that remained and restored vision to the affected mice.

These kinds of studies are important in developing the therapies of the future. Using mice in this way enabled researchers to discover precisely which stage of photoreceptor cell development could provide a renewable source of cells for effective repair. Future work will build on this knowledge and hopefully will result in advances in regenerative medicine that will benefit patients suffering from photoreceptor cell loss.

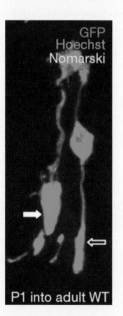

Figure 6.7 Transplanted retinal precursor cells become rods and cones. This micrograph shows two cells which were transplanted as retinal precursor cells into the retinas of adult mice. The cell on the left (filled arrow) has become a cone and the cell on the right (open arrow) has become a rod. It is possible to distinguish these donor cells from the host cells because the cells from the donor mouse are labelled with a fluorescent protein which makes them look green under the microscope. Magnification × 1000. (Source: MacLaren et al., 2006, Figure 1e).

6.4 Diabetic retinopathy

Diabetic retinopathy was added to the WHO Vision 2020 priority eye diseases list because it was becoming a major cause of sight loss in middle-income and developed countries. There were an estimated 135 million people in the world with diabetes in 1995 and 177 million in 2002 (WHO, 2004). The rate of increase in the incidence of diabetes is accelerating in the developed world.

People with diabetes develop persistent high blood pressure and high concentrations of blood glucose, which can gradually damage blood capillaries in the retina, a condition known as retinopathy. In its mildest form, the capillaries leak (they *haemorrhage*: Figure 6.8) but there is no effect on the individual's vision. The charity Diabetes UK estimates that one in four people with diabetes have retinopathy without experiencing any symptoms. This could be revealed by an eye test involving non-invasive examination of the retina.

Most sight loss due to diabetes can be prevented. At an early stage. the damaged capillaries can receive laser treatment to prevent further leakage. The high-intensity beam of light can be directed very precisely onto the retina and used to seal off the damaged vessels. However, laser treatment cannot restore lost vision nor will it affect the factors that are causing damage to the vessels. Those problems have to be dealt with separately, by gaining better control of blood pressure and the levels of glucose circulating in the blood.

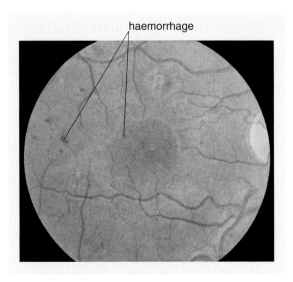

haemorrhage

Figure 6.8   Image of a damaged retina showing haemorrhages. (Source: Dr Renee Page)

A green-coloured Argon ion laser is used for treatment of diabetic retinopathy rather than the ultraviolet laser used in LASIK treatment. The aim is to destroy the leaky blood vessels that have developed over the retina by a *photothermal* process – that is, the light energy of the laser is directly converted into heat energy in order to raise the temperature of the vessels enough to destroy them.

The green laser light used is in the visible range of the electromagnetic spectrum, and so can travel through the cornea to the retina without hindrance.

◆ If the laser light is green, what colour pigment will absorb it? (Refer back to Figure 3.4.)

◆ Green is absorbed by the red and blue ends of the spectrum, i.e. reddish brown colours – the colour of blood.

The wavelength of laser light is chosen to match the wavelength at which blood absorbs the greatest number of photons (580 nm, green). This ensures heating of the blood vessels while avoiding heating other tissues in the beam. This heating destroys the cells within the vessel walls, and also makes the blood within the vessels solidify (or 'coagulate'). This coagulation seals both ends of the vessel and prevents later bleeding into the vitreous humour of the eye.

◆ What are the differences between the laser treatments used in LASIK and diabetic retinopathy?

◆ These lasers emit photons of different wavelengths, in the UV and visible ranges respectively. Also laser treatment for diabetic retinopathy aims to heat tissue (photothermal process) while LASIK light breaks chemical bonds without heating.

If the early stages of retinopathy are not detected, further deterioration occurs.

◈ What will happen if the macula becomes damaged?

◆ Once the macula becomes damaged, central vision will be affected.

Not everyone is affected in the same way, because it depends on precisely which area of the macula is damaged. It might be that vision is blurred or fuzzy when looking at an object close to the eye; for example, reading may be impaired. Or it may become difficult to see the detail of a face in the distance and thus be hard to recognise friends. In general, people do not lose all their functional sight at this stage, nor does everyone who has diabetes develop eye problems, but the longer one has diabetes the greater the risk (see Vignette 6.2) because, with this condition, it is rarely possible to avoid complications with the circulatory system.

There is, however, a more serious condition known as *proliferative retinopathy* that can result in loss of vision and can occur very suddenly. There is increased growth of new blood vessels in the retina (i.e. the vessels proliferate). This new growth is a response to a failing blood supply to the retina that has come about as a result of blood vessels becoming blocked. Unfortunately the new vessels often grow in the wrong places, preventing light from falling onto the sensory cells of the retina, the rods and cones. The vessels also tend to be weak and they bleed frequently, often severely. Bleeding into the vitreous humour impairs vision because the blood is opaque. Although the blood is gradually reabsorbed once the bleeding stops, the repair of the vessels involves formation of scar tissue that can pull the retina away from the pigmented epithelial cells. This is known as retinal detachment. If retinal detachment is not treated quickly the rods and cones die and vision is lost for ever.

The symptoms of a retinal detachment include flashes of light in the peripheral vision and the sensation that a curtain is falling across the eye. It is an emergency situation requiring immediate surgery to force the retina to lie back onto the pigment cells. Diabetic retinopathy is only one of a number of conditions that can lead to retinal detachment. However, since it is known that people with diabetes are at risk of developing eye problems, they should have regular eye examinations, together with a prompt visit to the optician if any problems with vision occur, as a routine part of the management of the disease.

Of course, there are many parts of the world where the basic facilities that allow an individual the opportunity to manage their condition effectively, do not exist. However, it is distressing that even in countries that do offer these facilities people are not taking advantage of them. For example, various estimates put the number of people with diabetes in the UK at around 3 million, of whom about 1 million are undiagnosed. Of those who know they have diabetes, roughly half do not have regular eye tests, thereby exposing themselves to unnecessary risk of visual impairment.

Vignette 6.2   Dave's story: Diabetes and blindness

Dave was diagnosed with diabetes aged 5 years old in the 1950s. He experienced no eye problems until he was 45 years old when retinopathy developed in both eyes. He describes this as: *Areas of darkness, sprinkly lights*. Despite laser treatment he lost a large area of sight in his left eye. He says: *It is a light-grey cup-shaped area where light is sensed by the eye but I cannot discern any image*. Now (2008) Dave has lost all vision in his left eye and peripheral vision in his right eye. He is registered blind and admits to feeling vulnerable in crowds and at road crossings. He also feels irritated at his loss of independence (made far worse in his case because he is also deaf and lip reads). He describes here how he copes:

Having been an avid reader I find my eye gets tired very quickly so I use a fluorescent lamp (supplied by the RNIB) which means I can read for longer. For me, bright light hurts the inside of the eye and dim light is an 'uncomfortable' struggle. Watching TV is great; I can really concentrate because the only thing in my vision is the screen. Whilst watching TV, I wear wrap-around plastic dark-blue glasses which are designed to block out light from all other angles. These are supplied by the RNIB as is my large-face, high-contrast wrist-watch. In my flat I know where EVERYTHING is and I never have cups or glasses anywhere near the edge of a table. Support rails in my shower are positioned so it is more difficult to fall. They are dark blue against contrasting matt tiles to avoid glare. As many surfaces as possible are non-glare and as far as possible I avoid bright white pages or paper. I have a red and white sturdy cane with rotating ball to help avoid obstacles and find kerbs, changes in floor materials, heights of steps. The cane also tells me the nature of the material as the vibrations travel up to my hand, so I can distinguish between slippery marble and rough concrete. I never tackle steps or stairs without a handrail unless supported by someone, as the chances of falling are high.

Recently Dave, who was a popular Open University tutor, has been given a computer by his friends who want to stay in touch but cannot telephone him because of his deafness. Email is allowing him to communicate more widely than before (Figure 6.9) but having lost his sight late in life and with multiple disabilities, he finds life more of a struggle than does Derek whom you met in Chapter 1.

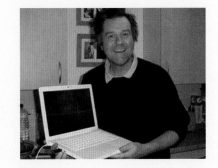

Figure 6.9   Dave's computer improves his ability to communicate with friends. (Source: Julian Miller)

Now would be a good time to study Activity 6.1 which considers global inequalities in accessibility of treatment for chronic eye conditions.

Activity 6.1   Global inequalities in eye treatment

Allow 20 minutes

Treatable visual impairments are common in poor communities around the world, causing long-term disadvantage in education and employment. This video on the DVD associated with this book shows eye tests, spectacles and cataract surgery provided at low cost to rural populations in South Africa and Southern India by 'health trains' that reach people in remote areas. You will see a cataract operation on the Indian train and in an English hospital, using similar procedures to insert a replacement lens. But some sight-saving treatments which are commonplace in the UK, such as laser eye surgery to treat diabetic retinopathy, are too costly for many people in developing countries.

Some of the videos show actual eye surgery and some of you may be uncomfortable viewing surgical procedures.

6.5   Eye infections

So far in this chapter, we have concentrated on chronic structural causes of visual impairment. Now we explore problems that can occur following interactions with **pathogens** (disease-causing organisms), particularly bacteria. **Bacteria** are small organisms that come in two basic shapes: spheres of approximately 1 μm (10^{-6} m) in diameter, and rods measuring around 1 μm by 3–4 μm (Figure 6.10). Bacteria are everywhere around us, and live in and on us too. Our bodies comprise about 10^{12} cells, but the number of bacteria associated with each of us is about 10^{14}; that is, there are 100 times more bacterial cells than human cells in each human body! Most of these bacteria live in our gut, where they help digestion and the passage of food through the bowel. Bacteria grow well on surfaces like the skin, and some take the opportunity to enter the body through wounds, causing infections. Bacteria on our bodies are usually kept in check by defence mechanisms such as antibacterial molecules in sweat and tears, and the 'sweeping' of the eye's surface caused by blinking. The vast majority have no effect on us at all, and many, like the gut bacteria just mentioned, are positively helpful. However, a tiny minority of pathogenic bacteria can cause us harm.

Remember that 10^{-6} is the scientific way of writing 0.000 001.

One notable feature of bacteria is that they can multiply very quickly. They do so by growing to twice their original size, then dividing into two. Each daughter bacterium repeats the process, so numbers double at each division. Growth and division processes are affected by temperature: bacteria that live on human bodies enjoy the warmth that we provide, and grow less quickly at lower temperatures. In ideal conditions some bacteria can double in numbers every 20 minutes. The rapid division rate that bacteria can achieve means that a small initial number of bacteria can reach huge numbers within a very short time. Thus the body's defences are adapted to removing harmful bacteria from the body as quickly as possible, as well as neutralising their effects by other means.

◆ Suggest some ways in which bacteria can be ejected from the body.

◆ Coughing, sneezing, vomiting, diarrhoea, crying.

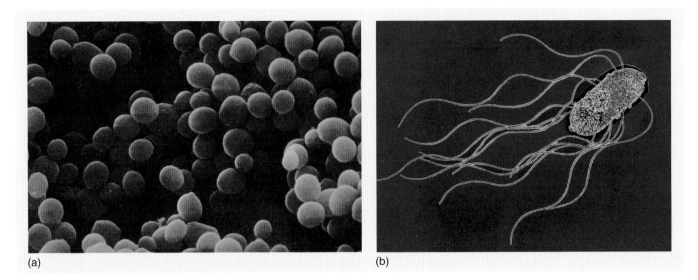

(a)

(b)

Figure 6.10 Microscopic appearance of bacteria: (a) spheroid (magnification × 2750) (Source: David M. Phillips/ Visual Sun Limited); (b) rod-shaped (magnification × 6500). (Source: Dr Linda Stannard, UCT/Science Photo Library)

6.5.1 Bacteria and the eye

One of the surfaces of our bodies that is vulnerable to pathogen attack is the outer surface of the eye. The eye has good defences against bacteria, particularly tears that flow over the surface, washing most bacteria away before they have a chance to colonise the eye. Tears also contain a number of antibacterial molecules such as lysozyme, whose action bursts the bacteria. Dead bacteria are then cleared by blinking (Section 2.1).

In spite of these defences, sometimes infections become established on and around the eye. Most people are familiar with **conjunctivitis**, a set of symptoms resulting from inflammation of the conjunctiva, the thin sheet of cells covering the inside of the eyelids and overlying the cornea. Inflammation produces the red itchiness that is common among babies and children, and affects many adults too. There are many causes of conjunctivitis, including hay fever or other allergies, herpes virus infections, and irritating chemicals such as chlorine from swimming pools, but a major cause is infection by bacteria, especially *Chlamydia trachomatis* (Box 6.2). Bacterial conjunctivitis is highly **contagious**, meaning that it is readily passed on to another person by contact. This contact need not be physically eye-to-eye (which is actually rare), but by a more indirect route, such as eye – hand – cup – hand – eye. One reason that infections can be passed on in this way is that the bacteria readily stick to surfaces and multiply quickly. Just a light touch to an infected eye means that the hand can then be contaminated by millions of bacteria. Even if only a small percentage is transferred at each step, the next person's eye can still be infected with enough bacteria to initiate a new case of the disease. Conjunctivitis can be treated with antibiotics, which cure bacterial conjunctivitis but have no effect on conjunctivitis resulting from other causes. Nevertheless, all cases of conjunctivitis should be treated as though they were contagious, and children with the condition are generally excluded from nursery and day-care until the eye symptoms have subsided, as itchy eyes will be rubbed, and any infection can easily be passed on.

Growth of a bacterial population is described in the DVD associated with another book in this series, *Water and Health in an Overcrowded World* (Halliday and Davey, 2007).

◆ Taking the infection route eye – hand – hand – eye, and assuming 1% of the bacteria are transferred at each step, how many bacteria will be transferred to the second eye if one million bacteria contaminate the first hand?

◆ One hundred. One per cent of one million (10^6) is ten thousand (10^4), and these bacteria are transferred to the second hand. This hand transfers 1% of ten thousand, i.e. one hundred (10^2) bacteria to the second eye.

Box 6.2 (Explanation) How organisms are named in biology

Chlamydia trachomatis provides an example of how organisms are named in biology. This naming system uses two Latin or Greek words, the first referring to a group of similar species, the second to one specific species. At least four species of *Chlamydia* are known, of which *Chlamydia trachomatis* is the best studied. Species names are always printed in italics and are often abbreviated, as in *C. trachomatis*.

6.5.2 Trachoma

Conjunctivitis caused by *C. trachomatis* is a common, unpleasant but relatively minor eye infection that is easily treatable with antibiotics applied as eye drops. The antibiotics kill the bacteria, stopping them multiplying and removing the source of infection. But if treatment is not available, the infection can become much more serious and result in the most globally important infectious eye disease of all: **trachoma**.

A scar is the mark produced by tissue healing, resulting from thickening of the area.

Figure 6.11 shows an advanced case of *C. trachomatis* infection. Following the red, itchy inflammation of the conjunctiva, the eye feels gritty and there is a thick discharge of tears, pus and bacteria. Paradoxically, tear production slows, so bacteria are less easily washed out. Because the eye is less well lubricated than usual, and the cornea and eyelids become red and sore, closing the eye becomes difficult. As the eye is rubbed, scarring occurs on the eyelids. This causes them to grow inwards, and the eyelashes rub against, and grow into, the cornea, causing scarring on the eye itself.

The ingrowing of the eyelashes, called **trichiasis** (trick-eye-ass-iss), is excruciatingly painful – think how much it hurts when one eyelash gets stuck in your eye. The irritation can lead to further infections and ulcers (damage to the surface, producing more soreness and pus) on the eye. The resulting scarring leads to blindness as scar tissue grows across the pupil, interfering with the passage of light into the eye and the ability of the cornea to focus it. Once the infection has reached this stage, eyesight cannot be restored even if the infection is eliminated as the scar tissue is permanent, so it is important to treat the disease as early as possible with antibiotics.

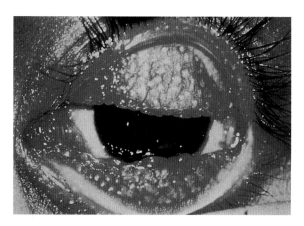

Figure 6.11 An eye affected with trachoma, showing extensive scarring of the conjunctiva. (Source: Armed Forces Institute of Pathology)

Most cases of trachoma occur in children, and infections easily pass between them as they play together, and to the adults who care for them. Although people acquire resistance to infections they have suffered before, eyes are particularly prone to repeated infections by the same organism because the outer parts of the eye are effectively 'outside' the body, and not in close contact with circulating blood which carries defence molecules. Each time a trachoma infection occurs, some scarring may result, and over time the repeated infections can result in trichiasis. Scarring usually appears in the twenties, and trichiasis in the forties, in people who have been repeatedly infected.

Vignette 6.3 describes how trachoma can affect people.

Vignette 6.3   Mzurisana's story

Mzurisana is a 45-year-old Maasai woman living in rural Tanzania (Figure 6.12). She suffers from blinding trachoma. The infection spreads through contact with eye discharge from an infected person on towels, handkerchiefs, fingers and flies. Poor hygiene, crowded households, water shortages and flies fuel its spread through the family and the community.

Mzurisana waited five years before seeking treatment for her pain and deteriorating vision.

'I couldn't afford the bus fare or the time away from my work to go and have surgery at the hospital', she explains. 'Instead, I used tweezers to pluck the eyelashes that were rubbing against my eyes and causing the pain'.

She wasn't aware that she was only worsening her situation by making her lashes shorter and sharper. Mzurisana finally went for the surgery that she needed to stop the progression of the disease, but it was too late to save her eyesight.

'Since having the surgery, things have been a little easier, but I still can't see very well.'

Before trachoma affected her eyesight, Mzurisana made and sold bead necklaces. With the income she was able to buy food and other essentials for her family. Today, Mzurisana cannot see well enough to make necklaces. She survives on the little money she earns by selling milk and by borrowing food from neighbours. She cannot afford to send her children to school.

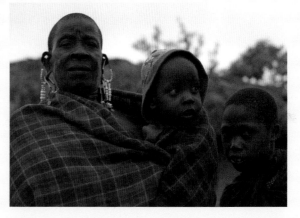

Figure 6.12   Mzurisana and two of her children. (Source: WHO/ Chris de Bode)

Mzurisana's plight could have been prevented by better community education about eye health and more accessible healthcare services. Surgery would have saved her eyesight if she had had it earlier.

WHO has set a global goal to eliminate blinding trachoma by the year 2020 as part of the Vision 2020 programme (see Section 6.5.3). Substantial progress has already been made, but sustained efforts are necessary to ensure that the next generation does not suffer from this preventable chronic disease.

More than ten countries across several regions of the world are on track to eliminate this disease forever.

In the developed world treatment is readily available and few cases of blindness result from *C. trachomatis* infection. But in the worst hit areas, in Africa and Asia, the statistics are horrifying, as shown in Table 6.1.

Table 6.1 Global incidence of trachoma. (Source: WHO, 2007c)

Condition	Number of people (millions)
living in countries where trachoma is endemic, so at risk of blinding trachoma	590
active trachoma	84
trichiasis	11
blind from infection	8

◆ Suggest why people living in poor, hot and dusty environments are so vulnerable to the development of trachoma.

◆ Poor areas often have overcrowded populations, with increased opportunities for contact with infected people or objects. Hot areas are often short of clean water, so the ability to practise good hygiene is limited. Furthermore, the high environmental temperature favours the growth of bacteria. Dusty environments suggest again a shortage of water; also dust particles blow into eyes, causing additional irritation and eye rubbing, and further damaging the conjunctiva.

6.5.3 Preventing trachoma blindness

Trachoma is a *preventable* cause of blindness. The organisation Sightsavers International contributes to the WHO programme *Vision 2020: The Right to Sight* with a programme for the global elimination of trachoma by 2020, and has developed a strategy called **SAFE**. This stands for **S**urgery, **A**ntibiotics, **F**acial cleanliness and **E**nvironmental change. Surgery is an effective way of treating trichiasis, removing scarred tissue from the eyelids and restoring them to their normal shape, getting the eyelashes out of the eyes. Surgery can reduce pain, and improves the quality of life of people with trachoma. As mentioned above, antibiotics kill the bacteria and remove the cause of the infection, allowing the body to heal itself and restore good eye function such as tear production. Facial cleanliness involves frequent face and hand washing in clean water, washing away dirt, bacteria and infectious eye secretions. It also makes the eyes less attractive to flies, which are strongly attracted to watery, salty secretions like tears.

◆ Why is it important to discourage flies?

◆ If a fly lands on an infected eye, it picks up *C. trachomatis*, which it transmits to the next eye that it lands on, passing on the cause of the disease.

Environmental change encompasses several issues. Above all, water supplies must be safe and clean. This may mean sinking boreholes well away from effluent sources like latrines, or may involve other 'point of use' strategies, such as filtration through cloth or use of water purification chemicals. People are

If you are studying this book as part of an Open University course, turn to Activity C1 in the *Companion* now.

The importance of clean water is discussed in another book in the series (Halliday and Davey, 2007).

reluctant to 'waste' scarce clean water on washing rather than drinking, but some compromise can be reached by the use of a 'leaky tin' (Figure 6.13), which allows faces and hands to be showered with a relatively small amount of water. Using soap removes dirt and also helps to kill bacteria.

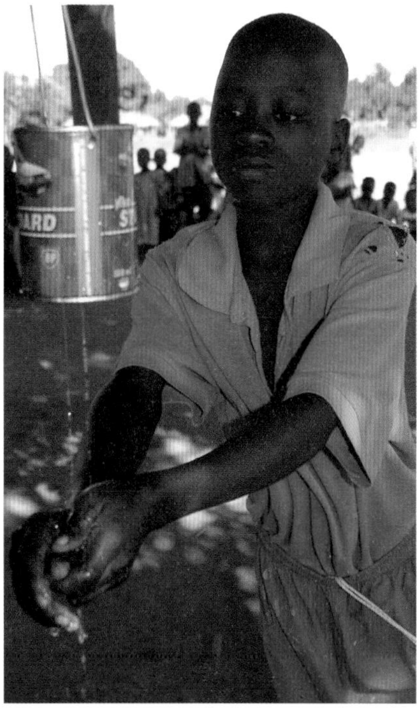

◆ Can you suggest another useful environmental change?

◆ Measures should be taken to discourage flies.

Flies are attracted by salty secretions, as you saw above. These include animal sweat, and livestock and their droppings provide a place for flies to live and breed. It is common in many African and Asian communities for people to live in close proximity with their livestock, even though it means that they are plagued by more flies. Education and provision of sound fencing (to prevent theft, straying and predation of the animals) are practical measures to reduce exposure to flies. Latrines also attract flies, and one way to reduce this particular problem is to cover the latrines, restricting fly access (Figure 6.14). There may be cultural hurdles to achieving this, but education and practical help can go a long way. The biggest barrier to provision of covered latrines is the money required to build them.

Figure 6.13 Using a leaky tin for washing when water is scarce. (Source: Jenny Matthews/ Sightsavers International)

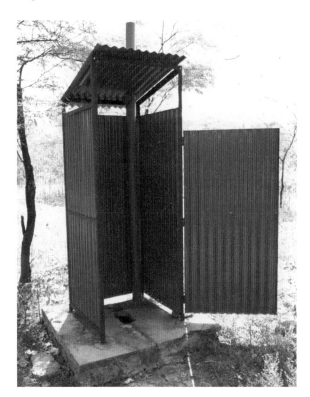

Figure 6.14 A covered latrine in Peru. 2.4 billion people worldwide do not have access to even this basic level of sanitation. (Source: WHO/HPR/TDR/Crump)

6.6   The big picture: clean water and the human condition

As you near the end of this book, we invite you to reflect on visual impairment in a wider context. We do not live in isolation on planet Earth, but in a dynamic balance both with the physical environment and with other inhabitants of the planet, be they other human beings, flies, livestock or bacteria. What can be learned about this balance from the example of trachoma? Here are some points to consider, but they do not constitute the whole list of issues, and no doubt you can think of more.

1   Every organism has its own set of preferred environmental conditions. Trachoma is a disease caused by bacteria that are adapted to live in our eyes.

2   *C. trachomatis* is a well-adapted pathogen: it encourages behaviour that can result in its spread (itching and consequent eye-rubbing), and it does not kill its host in the short term.

3   The occurrence and severity of trachoma infection depends on a balance between physical factors (temperature, water availability), biological factors (human population density, proximity of livestock, number of flies, presence of *C. trachomatis*), and social factors (availability of eye healthcare, education about disease prevention).

4   Trachoma is a preventable cause of visual impairment, and the SAFE strategy highlights physical, biological and social measures to eliminate it. None of them is beyond our capabilities, but economic and cultural difficulties may impede progress.

5   Fundamental to the susceptibility of a population to trachoma infection is the availability of clean water. When water is plentiful, good hygiene practices can be maintained, preventing the occurrence and spread of this, and many other diseases. A lack of clean water leads inexorably to a low quality of life, poor nutrition, and spread of disease.

At the time of writing (2008), more than 1 billion people across the world live without access to clean water for drinking and washing. It is little wonder, then, that many risk infection by *C. trachomatis* and other pathogens. This message needs to be taken seriously, and the political will generated to give everybody this bare necessity of life.

Summary of Chapter 6

6.1   Cataract, globally the leading cause of blindness, is caused by deterioration of lens proteins. However, cataract surgery is a relatively inexpensive and successful treatment.

6.2   Raised intraocular pressure leads to glaucoma, of which there are several types. By definition, they all lead to damage of the optic nerve. Damage to the optic nerve cannot be repaired. Damage can go unnoticed for some time because the brain 'fills in' for 'holes' in the visual field. Once detected, the progression of the condition can be arrested by appropriate medication. Treatment must be continuous and for life.

6.3   Although uncommon, closed-angle glaucoma can present as an acute episode leading to sudden loss of sight.

6.4   In age-related macular degeneration (AMD) the retinal blood vessels deteriorate, leading to death of the rods and cones because their supplies of oxygen and nutrients are inadequate and waste products are not removed. There is no cure for AMD but it progresses slowly, painlessly and rarely leads to complete loss of sight.

6.5   The rarer and more serious condition of wet AMD can be arrested by laser surgery to seal leaky blood vessels.

6.6   Diabetes, a chronic condition where raised blood pressure and blood glucose levels lead to leaking or over-growing blood vessels (diabetic retinopathy), can cause visual impairment with consequences for quality of vision that are similar to those of AMD. The detrimental effects can be reduced using laser treatment.

6.7   Eyesight can be affected not just by structural defects, but also by infections. The most common eye pathogen is the bacterium *Chlamydia trachomatis*. It infects millions of people worldwide. *C. trachomatis* causes conjunctivitis, but when left untreated the infection can progress to trachoma, with trichiasis and blindness ensuing.

6.8   Trachoma is a preventable disease, and there is a programme to eliminate it by 2020. The plan of action is the SAFE strategy – surgery, antibiotics, facial cleanliness and environmental change. Freedom from eye infections depends fundamentally on the availability of clean water.

Learning outcomes for Chapter 6

After studying this chapter and its associated activities, you should be able to:

LO 6.1   Define and use in context, or recognise definitions and applications of, each of the terms printed in **bold** in the text. (Questions 6.1, 6.2 and 6.3)

LO 6.2   Describe the causes, risk factors, treatments and preventative measures for the chronic conditions of cataract, glaucoma, AMD and diabetic retinopathy. (Question 6.2)

LO 6.3   Explain how some chronic eye conditions are diagnosed and the benefits of regular eye tests. (Question 6.3)

LO 6.4   Describe the possible impact of visual impairment on an individual. (Question 6.3 and Activity C1 in the *Companion*)

LO 6.5   Describe the role of *Chlamydia trachomatis* in eye infections. (Question 6.1 and Activity C1 in the *Companion*)

LO 6.6   List the routes by which *C. trachomatis* can be transmitted from one person to another. (Question 6.1 and Activity C1 in the *Companion*)

LO 6.7   Explain the importance of clean water in the prevention of eye infections. (Question 6.4 and Activity C1 in the *Companion*)

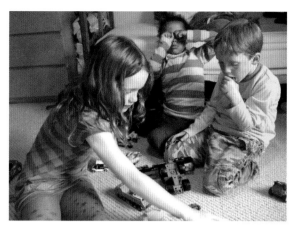

Figure 6.15 Small children playing together. (Source: Abi Davey)

Self-assessment questions for Chapter 6

If you are studying this book as part of an Open University course, you have also had the opportunity to demonstrate LOs 6.4, 6.5, 6.6 and 6.7 by completing Activity C1 in the *Companion*.

Question 6.1 (LOs 6.1, 6.5 and 6.6)

Look at Figure 6.15 and suggest ways in which an infection with *C. trachomatis* might be transmitted between the children. If they were playing in an area where trachoma is common, how might flies be involved in transmitting the infection?

Question 6.2 (LOs 6.1 and 6.2)

Distinguish between open-angle and closed-angle glaucoma and say which ethnic groups are particularly at risk from each of these eye diseases.

Question 6.3 (LOs 6.1, 6.3 and 6.4)

How might the treatment and prognosis for an individual experiencing sudden pain, headache and nausea with blurred vision be affected by where they live, and how might the situation have been averted?

Question 6.4 (LO 6.7)

Give one example of a barrier to using clean water to minimise eye infections and suggest a possible solution.

ANSWERS AND COMMENTS

Answers to self-assessment questions

Question 1.1

A cataract is a clouding of the lens of the eye, which prevents light from passing through it. The majority of cataracts are age-related and occur after the age of 50, but they can also develop following an eye injury and children are at greatest risk of this occurring.

Question 1.2

They are: (1) failure of the healthcare services to detect, intervene and treat preventable blindness soon enough; (2) inequalities in access to education and training for employment among people with severe visual impairments; (3) inadequate funding and provision of support and services to enable blind and partially sighted people to achieve greater independence; and (4) the right to aids that support reading, to empower people through access to the knowledge they need to improve their lives.

Question 1.3

People who live in impoverished circumstances are more at risk of developing a visual impairment through accident, injury or environmental factors such as infection, or exposure to irritants such as smoke from indoor cooking fires or pollutants. They are also the least able to access treatment and supportive services. Sight loss pushes them (and often their families) further into poverty because they are less able to earn a living and fulfil the functions of normal daily life – so visual impairment exacerbates poverty and vice versa, in a 'vicious cycle'.

Question 2.1

A person with a detached retina will no longer have light-sensitive retinal cells at the position where a sharp image is formed within the eyeball. As a result, vision will be blurred.

Question 2.2

The insect will elicit a blink reflex which protects the cornea of the eye. Tears will also be produced which remove any dirt or microbes that may remain in the eye.

Question 2.3

Ultraviolet light has a greater frequency (and shorter wavelength) than visible light, as shown in Figure 2.5.

Question 2.4

(a) The pupil is the opening at the front of the eye and determines the amount of light entering the eye. (b) The sclera prevents other extraneous light from transmission through the eyeball; (c) The retina is the light-sensitive tissue onto which an image is projected at the back of the eye.

Question 2.5

Your lens must accommodate to keep the train in focus. As the train moves further into the distance, the lens of the eye must become progressively thinner to maintain focus. This effect is produced by the ciliary muscles relaxing and allowing the suspensory ligaments to be pulled taut, flattening the curvature of the lens.

Question 2.6

The pigment melanin absorbs this light in the choroid and RPE. This is important because otherwise light rays would reflect within the eye creating extra images (or extra parts of an image) on the retina – like the double exposure effect on camera film where a second photograph overlays the first.

Question 2.7

The occipital lobe, which contains the primary visual cortex, is situated at the back of the brain. There is the possibility that the person's vision could be affected by an injury to that part of the brain. This may be permanent or temporary, depending on the exact location and degree of brain damage.

Question 3.1

When an object appears to a viewer to be white then *all* the visible light is reflected and none is absorbed.

Question 3.2

The unripe tomato absorbs more red wavelengths and reflects more green than the ripe tomato in Figure 3.3.

Question 3.3

(a) The complementary colour to orange is blue, so orange objects absorb blue light. (b) Blood is red and so absorbs the green-blue colour called cyan. (c) Blue objects absorb orange wavelengths.

Question 3.4

Figure 3.9 shows that both the green (M) and red (L) cones will be stimulated and that the mixture will be interpreted by the brain as an orangey-yellow colour.

Question 3.5

In this case, green and red can be distinguished but blue cannot be distinguished from red or green.

Question 4.1

6/18 vision means the individual could see at 6 metres what 'normal' sighted people can at 18 metres. Therefore I have myopia, as I cannot see objects far away.

Question 4.2

Looking at Figure 4.2, myopia occurs because sharp images form in front of the retina, in the vitreous humour.

Question 4.3

The camera was not focused properly during the photograph. The optical power of the camera lens was not the value needed to form a sharp image at the position of the film.

Question 4.4

Using Equation 4.2 relating focal length to optical power:

$$\text{focal length (m)} = \frac{1}{\text{optical power (D)}} = \frac{1}{66 \text{ D}} = 0.015 \text{ m}$$

The focal length is 0.015 m or 1.5 cm.

Question 4.5

Using Equation 4.3 for the combined optical power of two lenses.

$$D_{\text{TOTAL}} = D_1 + D_2 \qquad\qquad (4.3)$$

You know that $D_{\text{TOTAL}} = 66$ D and the optical power of the cornea, $D_1 = 59$ D, so you can find D_2, the optical power of the eye lens:

$$66 \text{ D} = 59 \text{ D} + D_2$$

Rearranging:

$$D_2 = 66 \text{ D} - 59 \text{ D} = 7 \text{ D}$$

A 59 D cornea needs a 7 D eye lens for an overall optical power of 66 D.

Question 4.6

If I wear spectacles with concave lenses I am short-sighted. The optical power of concave lenses is negative and corrects for short-sighted eyes that have excessive optical power, as shown in DVD Activity 4.1.

Question 5.1

The laser eye surgeon can apply more laser pulses at the centre of the cornea. This ensures that more tissue is removed from the centre of the cornea than from the outer regions. The reduced curvature of the cornea corrects for short-sightedness.

Question 5.2

There are 100 centimetres in a metre. To convert metres into centimetres, you multiply by 100. Note that 100 can be written as 10^2 (as explained in Section 2.2).

1 centimetre, cm, is 1×10^{-2} m;
1 micrometre, μm, is 1×10^{-6} m.

One pulse removes 0.25 μm (or 0.25×10^{-6} m) of cornea tissue.

This can be expressed in centimetres as:

$$0.25 \times 10^{-6} \times 100 \text{ cm}$$

$$= 0.25 \times 10^{-6} \times 10^2 \text{ cm}$$

Looking back to Activity 2.1, this is rewritten as:

$$= 0.25 \times 10^{(-6+2)} \text{ cm}$$

$$= 0.25 \times 10^{-4} \text{ cm}$$

100 pulses removes $100 \times 0.25 \times 10^{-4}$ cm.

$$= 25 \times 10^{-4} \text{ cm}$$

$$= 2.5 \times 10^{-3} \text{ cm } (0.0025 \text{ cm})$$

20 pulses removes $20 \times 0.25 \times 10^{-4}$ cm

$$= 5.0 \times 10^{-4} \text{ cm } (0.0005 \text{ cm})$$

Question 5.3

The H----O hydrogen bond is weaker and longer than the O—H covalent bond in hydroxyl groups (see Figure 5.9).

Question 6.1

Infection from one of the children is likely to be transmitted by the following routes:

- Bacteria may be transferred from the infected eye of a child onto that child's hand, or onto a towel or other object such as a toy. When another child touches the infected towel, toy or hand, bacteria can pass onto their own hand, and thence onto their eyes if the eyes are rubbed or touched.

- Bacteria from an infected eye could be picked up on the feet of flies feasting on the watery pus in and around the eye. When the fly lands on the eye of the next child, the bacteria drop off the fly into the favourable environment of a fresh, uninfected eye, where they can multiply and cause disease.

Question 6.2

In both open-angle and closed-angle glaucoma, the drainage angle becomes blocked preventing fluid from leaving the aqueous cavity and leading to raised intraocular pressure, but the cause of the blockage differs in each case. In open-angled glaucoma the trabeculae silt up, whilst in closed-angle glaucoma the drainage angle closes because the iris and cornea become too close to one another. Africans are at particular risk from open-angle glaucoma and the Chinese are at particular risk from closed-angle glaucoma.

Question 6.3

These are symptoms of rapidly increasing intraocular eye pressure (an acute episode of closed-angle glaucoma). Medical attention needs to be given immediately to reduce eye pressure, and for people living in remote areas far from emergency medical treatment centres the chance of getting help before they lose their sight is poor. Regular eye tests can identify individuals who are at risk, although acute events cannot be predicted.

Question 6.4

The most important environmental factor in trachoma prevention is the availability and use of clean water. In many parts of the world, particularly where trachoma is endemic, clean water is in very short supply. People are therefore unwilling to use water for washing, when they could instead use it for drinking. One solution to this is to use a leaky tin which provides a shower of water for washing hands and faces. Sources of effluent must be kept away from supplies of clean water, and one way to do this is to use latrines, but there may be cultural and educational issues surrounding the use of these structures.

Comments on activities

Activity 2.1

Example calculation: calculating the wavelength of orange light

For orange light, the wave frequency is approximately 5×10^{14} Hz or s^{-1}.

The speed of light in air is 3×10^8 m s^{-1}.

Equation 2.4 is used to calculate the wavelength from the speed and frequency values.

$$\text{wavelength (m)} = \frac{\text{speed (m s}^{-1})}{\text{frequency (Hz or s}^{-1})} \qquad (2.4)$$

$$\text{wavelength (m)} = \frac{3 \times 10^8 \text{ m s}^{-1}}{5 \times 10^{14} \text{ s}^{-1}}$$

This equation can be simplified by considering separately the number and the 'power of ten' components of each term:

$$\text{wavelength (m)} = \frac{3}{5} \times \frac{10^8}{10^{14}}$$

which is the same as

$$\text{wavelength (m)} = 0.6 \times \frac{10^8}{10^{14}}$$

$$\frac{10^8}{10^{14}} = 10^{(8-14)} = 10^{-6}$$

Therefore

wavelength (m) $= 0.6 \times 10^{(8-14)}$

wavelength (m) $= 0.6 \times 10^{-6}$

To convert from metres (m) to nanometres (10^{-9} m), you must multiply by 10^9.

wavelength $= (0.6 \times 10^{-6}) \times 10^9$ nm

wavelength $= 0.6 \times 10^{(-6+9)}$ nm

wavelength $= 0.6 \times 10^3$ nm

wavelength $= 600$ nm

The wavelength of orange light is 600 nm.

References

Brundtland, G. H. (2002) Speech on World Blindness Day, 9 October 2002. Available from: http://www.who.int/dg/brundtland/speeches/2002/en/ (Accessed November 2007)

CNIB symposium (2004) [online] A Clear Vision: Solutions to Canada's Vision Loss Crisis. Available from: http://www.cnib.ca/en/about/publications/research/ Default.aspx (Accessed November 2007)

Frick, K. D. and Foster, A. (2003) 'The magnitude and cost of global blindness: an increasing problem that can be alleviated', *American Journal of Ophthalmology*, vol. 135, no. 4, pp. 471–476.

Gilbert, C. and Foster, A. (2001) 'Childhood blindness in the context of Vision 2020 – The Right to Sight', *Bulletin of WHO 2001*, vol. 79, no. 3, pp. 227–232. [online] Available from: http://whqlibdoc.who.int/bulletin/ 2001/issue3/79(3)227-232.pdf (Accessed November 2007)

Gooding, K. (2006) *Poverty and Blindness: A Survey of the Literature*, a report for Sightsavers International, Haywards Heath, UK. Available from: http:// www.iceh.org.uk/files/poverty_and_blindess_02.06.pdf (Accessed August 2007)

Goss, D. A. (2000) 'Nearwork and myopia', *Lancet*, vol. 356, pp. 1456–1457.

Halliday, T. and Davey, B. (eds) (2007) *Water and Health in an Overcrowded World*, Oxford, Oxford University Press.

Hammond M. D., Madigan, W. P. Jr and Bower, K. S. (2005) 'Refractive surgery in the United States Army 2000–2003', *Ophthalmology*, vol. 112, pp. 184–190.

Jacobs, J. M., Hammerman-Rozenberg, R., Maaravi, Y., Cohen. A. and Stessman, J. (2005) 'The impact of visual impairment on health, function and mortality', *Aging Clinical and Experimental Research*, vol. 17, no. 4, pp. 281–286.

MacLaren, R. E., Pearson, R. A., MacNeil, A., Douglas, R. H., Salt, T. E., Akimoto, M., Swaroop, A., Sowden, J. C. and Ali, R. R. (2006) 'Retinal repair by transplantation of photoreceptor precursors', *Nature*, vol. 444, pp. 203–207.

McLaughlan (2006) [online] Open your Eyes, RNIB Campaign report. Available from: http://www.rnib.org.uk/xpedio/groups/public/documents/PublicWebsite/ public_oyereportword.doc (Accessed November 2007)

Midgley, C. A. (ed.) (2008) *Chronic Obstructive Pulmonary Disease: A Forgotten Killer*, Oxford, Oxford University Press.

Organisation of Economic Cooperation and Development (2005) *Health at a Glance: OECD Indicators 2005,* Organisation for Economic Cooperation and Development.

Orr, P., Barron, Y., Schein, O. D., Rubin, G. S. and West, S. K. (1999) 'Eye care utilisation by older Americans: the SEE project-Salisbury Eye Evaluation', *Ophthalmology*, vol. 106, no. 5, pp. 904–909.

Parvin, E. M. (ed.) (2007) *Screening for Breast Cancer*, Oxford, Oxford University Press.

Phillips, J. B. (ed.) (2008) *Trauma, Repair and Recovery*, Oxford, Oxford University Press.

Resnikoff, S., Pascolini, D., Etya'ale, D., Kocur, I., Pararajasegaram, R., Pokharel, G. P. and Mariotti, S. P. (2004) 'Global data on visual impairment in the year 2002', *Bulletin of the World Health Organisation*, vol. 82, no.11, pp. 844–851.

RNIB (2005) *Get the Picture*. Report on the campaign to make broadcasting accessible for people with sight problems, Royal National Institute for Blind People. Available from: http://www.rnib.org.uk/xpedio/groups/public/documents/code/InternetHome.hcsp (Accessed August 2007)

Sachdev, M. (2005) [online] The truth about spectacles. Available from: http://www.tribuneindia.com/2005/20050216/health.htm#1 (Accessed November 2007)

Sightsavers International [online] Available from: www.sightsavers.org (Accessed November 2007)

Smart, L. E. (ed.) (2007) *Alcohol and Human Health*, Oxford, Oxford University Press.

The Fred Hollows Foundation (2007) [online] Available from: http://www.hollows.org/ (Accessed November 2007)

Thornton, J., Edwards, R., Mitchell, P., Harrison, R. A., Buchan, I. and Kelly, S. P. (2005) 'Smoking and age-related macular degeneration: a review of association', *Eye*, vol. 19, pp. 935–944.

Toates, F. (ed.) (2007) *Pain*, Oxford, Oxford University Press.

Venkata, G., Murthy, S., Gupta, S.K., Bachani, D., Jose, R. and John, N. (2005) 'Current estimates of blindness in India', *British Journal of Ophthalmology*, vol. 89, pp. 257–260.

WHO (2004) Prevention of blindness and deafness: Diabetic retinopathy. Available from: www.who.int/pbd/blindness/vision_2020/priorities/en/index5.html (Accessed January 2006)

WHO (2006) Prevention of blindness and deafness: Refractive error and low vision. Available from: www.who.int/pbd/blindness/vision_2020/priorities/en/index5.html (Accessed January 2006)

WHO (2007a) Priority eye diseases. Available from: http://www.who.int/blindness/causes/priority/en/ (Accessed December 2007)

WHO (2007b) The Global Child Survival Partnership: a new initiative to save children's lives. Available from: http://www.who.int/child-adolescent-health/NEWS/news_35.htm (Accessed December 2007)

WHO (2007c) AFR/RC57/6 25 June 2007 [online] Regional Committee for Africa, 57th session, Brazzaville, Republic of Congo, 27–31 August 2007. *Accelerating the Elimination of Avoidable Blindness: A Strategy for the WHO African Region*. Available from: http://www.afro.who.int/rc57/documents/AFR-RC57-6_Elimination_of_Avoidable_Blindness_final.pdf (Accessed November 2007)

Useful websites, maintained by the OU Library through the ROUTES system (see 'About this book')

www.macular-degeneration.org [Macular Degeneration Network]

www.mayoclinic.com [Mayo Clinic]

www.rnib.org.uk [Royal National Institute of Blind People website]

www.afb.org [American Foundation for the Blind]

www.vao.org.uk [Vision Aid Overseas]

www.sightsavers.org.uk [Sightsavers International]

www.glaucoma-association.com [International Glaucoma Association]

ACKNOWLEDGEMENTS

Grateful acknowledgement is made to the following sources for permission to reproduce material in this book.

Figures

Figure 1.1: Phototake Inc/Photolibrary; Figure 1.2: WHO/Serge Resnikoff; Figure 1.3: Shezad Noohrani/Still Pictures; Figure 1.4: Jamshyd Masud/ Sightsavers International; Figures 1.5: Georgina Cranston/Sightsavers International; Figure 1.6: Derek Child; Figure 1.7: Tim Pohl/istockphoto;

Figure 2.4: Lesley Smart; Figure 2.16a: Biophoto Associates/Science Photo Library; Figure 2.17b: Joy Wilson/Boots Opticians;

Figure 3.1: John McGill; Figure 3.6a: Lesley Smart; Figure 3.7b: Gene Cox/ Science Photo Library; Figure 3.8 Accelrys;

Figure 4.3: Roger Courthold;

Figure 5.2b: David W. Hahn, http://plaza.ufl.edu/dwhahn; Figure 5.6: Science Museum/Science Photo Library; Figure 5.10: Jane Pang/istockphoto;

Figures 6.3, 6.4 and 6.12: WHO/Chris De Bode; Figure 6.7: MacLaren, R. E. et al. (2006) 'Retinal repair by transplantation of photoreceptor precursors', *Nature*, vol. 444, 9 November 2006, Macmillan Publishers Ltd; Figure 6.8: Dr Renee Page; Figure 6.9: Julian Miller; Figure 6.10a: David M. Phillips, Visual Sun Limited; Figure 6.10b: Dr Linda Stannard, UCT/Science Photo Library; Figure 6.11: Armed Forces Institute of Pathology; Figure 6.13: Jenny Matthews/ Sightsavers International; Figure 6.14: WHO/HPR/TDR/Crump; Figure 6.15: Abi Davey.

Every effort has been made to contact copyright holders. If any have been inadvertently overlooked the publishers will be pleased to make the necessary arrangements at the first opportunity.

INDEX

Entries and page numbers in **bold type** refer to key words which are printed in **bold** in the text. Indexed information on pages indicated by *italics* is carried mainly or wholly in a figure or a table.